THE TAO OF
Nutrition

By

MAOSHING NI, Ph.D., C.A.

With Cathy McNease, B.S., M.H.

Forward by Taoist Master Ni, Hua-Ching

Published by
The Shrine of the Eternal Breath of Tao
Malibu, California
and   ·
College of Tao and Traditional Chinese Healing
Mailing Address: 117 Stonehaven Way
                  Los Angeles, California 90049

Distributed by: Union of Tao and Man
                 117 Stonehaven Way
                 Los Angeles, CA 90049

Library of Congress Catalog Card
Number 87-60145

ISBN 0-937064-14-9

Printed in the U.S.A.

DEDICATION

"Eat not for the pleasure thou mayest find therein. Eat to increase thy strength. Eat to preserve the life thou has received from heaven."

Confucius

ACKNOWLEDGEMENT

I would like to express my deepest gratitude to my father who has endowed me with this great tradition and knowledge so that I may be able to share them with everyone. A special appreciation to Cathy McNease who untiringly transcribed all my lectures into readable form and helped to arrange and edit the text into this final version. Without her help, this book would not have become available. I would also like to thank all of my students, patients and friends for their valuable suggestions and feedback with the remedies in this book. To everyone who continues to support and promote natural medicine in this world, I am most grateful to all of you.

DISCLAIMER

This book is intended to present to the reader the energetic and the healing aspects of foods. It is the authors' desire to provide to those who are open minded about natural alternatives to healing. However, the remedies offered within are to the authors' best knowledge and experience and are to be used by readers at their own discretion. If you wish to try the therapeutic approaches outlined in this book for serious conditions, we advise you to find a doctor of oriental medicine that is familiar with the field of Chinese nutrition who can supervise you in your treatment program.

ABOUT THE AUTHORS

Maoshing Ni, born into a family of medical traditions as the thirty-eighth generation of traditional Chinese healers, began his training early in life. He studied intensively with his father, a Taoist Master and a Master healer, and many other teachers in the subjects of Chinese Medicine, martial arts, Tai Chi Chuan, Taoism and other related arts in China. He attended schools in China and the United States and received his advanced degrees and license as an acupuncturist. He is presently in private practice in Los Angeles and lectures extensively at acupuncture Colleges on various subjects of Chinese Medicine and dietary therapy. He also teaches Tai Chi Chuan and other energy exercises. His goal is to make Oriental Medicine widely available in the West, and someday, to see it not only as Oriental Medicine, but as universal medicine!

Cathy McNease is an herbalist and writer living in Ojai, California with her husband. Together they own a small Chinese herb business and teach classes in Taoism, herbalism, Chinese nutrition, and related subjects. She received degrees from Western Michigan University and Emerson College of Herbology and has studied under some of the most notable herbalists in this country. Much of her interest in nutrition began fifteen years ago when she first became a vegetarian and soon after purchased a natural food and herb store. For ten years she provided nutritional and herbal counselling at her store. Presently she contributes a regular column, "Cathy's Herb Corner", to a small wholistic journal, The Sharing News. As a student of the Ni family she continues to further her education in the Taoist healing arts.

TABLE OF CONTENTS

LIST OF RECIPES

FORWARD

The knowledge of nutrition in China has roots that go back at least 6,000 years and is based on the principles of balance and harmony, as well as direct knowledge of the nature of individual foods. This knowledge was first gathered by spiritually achieved men and women who, by their own experience, learned not only what properties specific foods contained, but also how to utilize them for the purposes of nutrition and longevity. Anyone who learns and uses this ancient, time-tested knowledge will find their health and longevity greatly enhanced.

Fu Shi, one of the great sages of ancient China, discovered eight categories of universal energy, which later came to be known as the "Ba Gua" or Eight Trigrams; this is a further division of the two main categories of natural energy known as yin and yang. The universe itself is an integration of these two interacting, mutually assisting and also somewhat opposing forces which are often expressed by the "Tai Chi" symbol illustrated on the front cover of this book. The deepest reality of universal life is the inner meaning of yin and yang, and, like yin and yang, the nature of the universe also tends to be both harmonious and balanced. Even events which could be conceptually classified as negative or conflicting, are only stages in the accomplishment of further harmonization. This is the truth expressed in the Tai Chi diagram.

Harmony and balance, therefore, the principles of universal existence, became the foundation of cultural development in ancient China and were widely applied in public and private life as well as in spiritual practice. Many generations later, whatever expressed these natural universal qualities of balance, harmony and symmetry came to be

i

known as "Taoism": Tao being the way or path of universal harmony through integration.

Shen Nung, another wise leader who lived some time after Fu Shi, used these principles to develop herbal medicine and essential nutrition. After him came the Yellow Emperor, one of the greatest leaders in human history, who has come to be considered the "founder" of Taoism. He further developed the contributions of the early sages, utilizing them in political as well as general life, especially in the realms of medicine and nutrition, and benefiting his hundred-year reign greatly by the guidance of this special knowledge.

Fu Shi, Shen Nung and the Yellow Emperor are great symbols of natural culture. Another symbolic figure of longevity is popular even now in Chinese culture. He is called Pung Tzu and is considered the founder of the art of Chinese cooking and nutrition. Pung Tzu learned all the arts of long life, including "Do-In", energy conducting exercises, and "Fang Zhong", the art and discipline of sexual practices. Pung Tzu is said to have lived to be 800 years old and was still active in the reign of the Emperor Jou, around 1123 B.C.

As the spiritual descendants of these men of spiritual development and dedication to human development, we can still benefit today from their great achievements and contributions, as many have done before us. Through the traditional Chinese healing arts and herbal medicine, I myself have offered much useful knowledge and help to many people around the world. Although I taught a class on diet and nutrition several years ago, there was still a secret wish in my mind to do more in this area. Because of my busy schedule, I have not had time to do so, but fortunately my son Maoshing had the same interest. Thus, he has brought this book into your hands to fill the gap in my own work. It can be an important and

ii

useful tool in your life that will serve your
health and spiritual development. With its
support, I wish that each of you may become
stronger every day.

Thank you,

Ni, Hua-Ching
January 1987
Los Angeles, CA.

PREFACE

In a rapidly changing society such as ours, people have lost their instinctive nature in the ways of eating. People have a poor concept of what makes up a good diet. They thrive and rely on their taste buds and visual sensations for sustenance. In most cases, they have not learned to eat to live, but rather live to eat. Even more sadly, caught in the daily rat race of their surroundings, many people take priority for work, pleasure, and sex over what they eat. Also, at the same time mind boggling numbers of different fads, cultists, and controversial dietary regimes add even more confusion to the already uncertain dietary habits of today's people.

All of these show in the deterioration of the quality of people's lives in modern society. The Tao of Nutrition presents the wisdom of the ancient Chinese. Ancient people were much more aware of the environment and how their bodies reacted to their surroundings. They lived by the principle of being in harmony with Nature and emphasized balance in every aspect of life, especially diet, the yin and yang of foods and of the body. Their knowledge and experiences were passed down through generations for many centuries, and further refined and systematized into what we call Chinese nutrition today.

The system of Chinese nutrition is a healing system of its own. Not only is it a healing system, but also a disease prevention system. The advantage of Chinese nutrition lies in its flexibility in adapting to every individual's needs, and treating the whole person instead of the disease.

Chinese nutrition differs from modern Western nutrition in that it does not rely on analyzing the chemical constituents of each food; rather, it

v

determines the properties or energies of each food and combination, taking into consideration season, method of preparation, and geographical location, and utilizes the information according to the natural principles of life and balance.

It is hoped that the readers of this book will gain insight and understanding into their bodies their surroundings, and their diet. So here it is, the essence of the science and the art of food. With this book in your hands you can be the master of your own body. Start now to better yourself and other people to achieve and maintain health, vitality, and longevity.

HOW TO USE THIS BOOK

This book contains three major sections: the first section deals with theories of Chinese nutrition and philosophy; the second section describes over 100 common foods in detail (their energetic properties, their therapeutic actions, and individual remedies); and the third section is a remedial section which gives recommendations for various medical conditions.

It is strongly recommended that readers familiarize themselves thoroughly with the first section in order to understand the basic philosophies of Chinese nutrition. With that understanding, one is able to more efficiently utilize the specific knowledge given in sections two and three.

Another way readers may find this book useful is to utilize it according to what condition may apply to them. So they may choose to look up a specific condition in the therapeutic remedies section and follow the recommendations given there. For example, if you look up "headache", you will find the following remedies to choose from:

For headaches due to common cold or flu:
1. Make tea from ginger and green onions, boiling for 5 minutes; drink and try to sweat.
2. Steam aching portion of head over mint and cinnamon tea that is cooking, then dry head afterwards, avoiding catching a draft.
3. Make tea from chrysanthemum flowers and cassia seeds and drink.
4. Make buckwheat meal into a paste and apply to painful area until it sweats.
5. Drink green tea.
6. Make rice porridge and add garlic and green onions. Eat while hot, then get under covers

and sweat.

For headaches due to high blood pressure,
menstrual cycles, emotional stress or tension, or
migraines:
1. Make carrot juice. If headache is on left side,
   squirt carrot juice into left nostril; if on
   right side, squirt into right nostril; if both
   sides are painful, squirt into both nostrils.
2. Take lemon juice and 1/2 T. baking soda mixed in
   a glass of water and drink.
3. Make tea of unripe green prunes, mint, and green
   tea.
4. Make tea of oyster shells and chrysanthemum
   flowers, boiling for 2 hours.
5. Mash peach kernels and walnuts, mix with rice
   wine and lightly roast it; take 2 T. 3 times
   daily.
6. Rinse head with warm water, gradually increasing
   the temperature to hot.

After studying the entire book, one will gain
an insight into maintaining balance and harmony
with one's body and environment and ultimately
achieve health, happiness and longevity.

SECTION

Introduction

Energetic Properties

Chinese nutrition is defined as "the science that deals with the healing properties of foods to correct disharmonies within the body." It differs from Western nutrition in that it does not talk about the biochemical nature of foods. Rather, Chinese nutrition deals on an energetic level to which balance is the key. Foods are selected according to their energetic qualities such as warming, cooling, drying, or lubricating. Thus, Chinese nutrition would seek to warm the coldness, cool the heat, dry the dampness, lubricate the dryness and so forth.

By carefully studying the individual's imbalances, one would choose the appropriate foods to bring about a balanced state of health. For example, for an excessive individual who is exhibiting conditions of heat in the body, cooling foods would be appropriate. For a deficient individual who tends toward coldness, warming foods would be chosen. In this way health is achieved. Foods all have specific qualities inherent within; then the method of preparation either enhances or neutralizes the foods. To make a food more cooling add liquid, sugar, honey, or fruit. To make a food more warming add heat, age, pressure, or salt. Generally speaking, warming foods raise metabolism and cooling foods lower metabolism.

Western nutrition, in general, is very mechanical and biochemical, measuring units of protein, carbohydrates, fats, vitamins, and minerals. One aspect that is worth mentioning is the acid-base (alkaline) balance. The pH is a measurement of this ratio. The scale goes from 1.0 (acid) to 14.0 (base); the human body should be on the alkaline side near 7.3. If the body's pH varies much away

5

from that there is discomfort or disease. The foods we eat contribute to the pH balance. In general, we want to consume a larger portion of alkaline foods (i.e. vegetables, fruits, millet, almonds, brazil nuts) and fewer acid foods (i.e. grains, beans, nuts, meats). Heavy meat eaters often tend to be too acidic, while vegetarians can easily tend towards being too alkaline. Balance within the diet is essential for good health.

Yin and Yang

It is a universal law that everything is constantly changing, except for the fundamental governing laws of life. This principle applies to the universe surrounding us as well as the inner universe of our bodies. The ancient Chinese developed ways of looking at these changes to better understand them. One such theory is that everything in the universe consists of two opposite yet complementary aspects. This is called the theory of yin and yang. Yin and yang exist relative to one another and are also in a state of change at any given time; they are not static conditions. Day and night are a good example of this. When yin and yang are out of balance diseases or disharmonies occur.

Within the body, yin and yang are often referred to as the body's water and fire. These descriptions are very useful in determining the relative nature of both the individual and the energies of foods. The application of Chinese nutrition necessitates determining the body type of the individual. He or she may be the *cold* type, considered of a yin nature, or the *hot* type, considered yang. Some significant questions to determine this may be as follows, with the yang tendencies listed first: male or female? feel hot or cold? drawn to hot or cold foods? thirst or no thirst? constipated or loose stools? dark or pale urine? red face or tongue or pale? We are all a mixture of yin and yang, although we may be predominantly one or the other. Thus, yang persons need relatively more yin (cooling) foods and yin types need relatively more yang (warming) foods.

Typical symptoms of the heat type or yang type person could include the following: red complexion, easy to sweat, always hot, dominating, aggressive or outgoing personality, coarseness, loud voice, dry mouth, thirst, ferocious appetite, constipation, foul breath, scanty and dark urine, sometimes dry cough with thick yellow sputum, easily angered, very emotional, early and heavy menstruation with bright red blood, irritability, and insomnia.

Typical symptoms of the cold type or yin type could include the following: paleness, coldness, drinks little fluids, low energy, loose stools, sleeps a lot, feeble and weak voice, introverted personality, white and copious sputum, lack of appetite, copious and clear urine, dizziness, and edema.

To bring about balance and counteract the symptoms, heat type persons would use primarily cooling foods such as fresh fruits, juices, and many of the vegetables. Cold type persons would achieve balance by regularly including the warming foods in their diet, such as garlic, ginger, green onions, black beans, sesame seeds, chicken, etc. Accordingly, heat types would avoid hot, spicy foods, while cold types would avoid cold, raw foods.

Yin and yang also apply to the organs of our

7

bodies. Those which are considered solid, or with much substance, are considered yin. These include heart, spleen, liver, lungs, kidneys. Those which are considered hollow, active in transportation, are considered yang. These include large and small intestines, gall bladder, stomach, and urinary bladder. Further descriptions of each organ will follow.

Five Elements

Another very useful theory in the Chinese view of the universe is the five elements theory or the five energy transformations. This gives us a helpful framework to understand the ever-changing world, the inner relationships of change, and the interconnectedness of all things. The five elements are Wood, Fire, Earth, Metal, and Water. You connect them in this sequence for what is called the creation cycle. This cycle occurs in nature as well as within our bodies. In nature, rub two pieces of wood together and create fire; fire burns to ash and becomes earth; from earth we dig up metal; melt the metal to liquid and make water; put a seed into the water and it germinates a tree and creates wood. It is a very circular cycle. (Refer to Chart 1.)

In the creation cycle the creator element is the mother who gives birth to the son element. Thus, if the son is weak or deficient, we can tonify (nourish) its mother and thereby benefit the son. In nature the five elements can be correlated to the seasons as follows: Wood corresponds to spring, Fire corresponds to summer, Earth corresponds to late summer, Metal corresponds to autumn, Water corresponds to winter.

In our body the organs are also referred to as

8

the elements. The correspondences are as follows: Wood is liver and gall bladder, Fire is heart and small intestines, Earth is spleen and stomach, Metal is lungs and large intestines, Water is kidneys and urinary bladder. So if there is not enough Fire, corresponding to the heart, we would strengthen the Wood organ, the liver, with the proper foods or herbs. In ancient times these correspondences were made by observing nature and how our bodies worked similarly. For example, the heart is probably the most active organ in the body. Also, when you fall in love it is said that your heart "burns with desire." Thus, the heart seems to closely correlate to the element of Fire.

There is a useful relationship between food colors and the elements and corresponding body systems. White foods nourish the lungs; black and dark blue foods nourish the kidneys; green foods nourish the liver; yellow and orange foods nourish the spleen-stomach; red foods nourish the heart. Thus, a person with weak digestion (spleen weakness) should include plenty of the yellow and orange foods, such as sweet potatoes and winter squashes, as these are the colors that correspond to the Earth element or the spleen organ. One with heart weakness would do well to eat more red foods such as tomatoes and hawthorn berries, as red corresponds to the element Fire and the organ the heart.

Another relationship that occurs within the five elements is the control cycle. (Refer to Chart 1.) It goes like this: we take wood, a tree, for example, whose roots invade into the earth; we take earth and build a dam to control water; water puts out the fire; fire melts down the metal; metal makes the ax that cuts the wood. If Wood (liver) becomes excessive, manifesting as hypertension, red

9

CHART 1 :

FIVE ELEMENTS (energetic transformation)

THE CREATION CYCLE

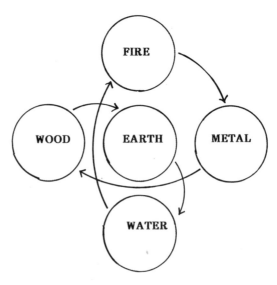

THE CONTROL CYCLE

CHART 2 :

THE CORRESPONDENCES OF
THE FIVE PHASES OF ENERGY EVOLUTION

FIRE

ORGANS:	HEART, SMALL INTESTINE, PERICARDIUM,
FLAVOR:	BITTER TRIPLE WARMER
SENSE:	TASTE-TONGUE
COLOR:	RED
EMOTION:	JOY
VOICE:	LAUGHTER
PHYSICAL MANIFESTATION:	VESSELS
MODE OF ACTION:	ITCHING
INTERNAL ENERGY:	SHEN CHI (DIRECTING ENERGY)
PHYSICAL ESSENCE:	MARROW
CLIMATE:	HEAT
DEVELOPMENT:	GROWTH
NEGATIVE DRIVE:	GREED
POTENTIALLY CORRUPTING INFLUENCE:	SEX
ATTRIBUTES OF MIND:	SPIRITUALITY
MORAL:	HUMILITY

METAL

LUNGS, LARGE INTESTINE
HOT
SMELL-NOSE
WHITE
SADNESS
CRYING
SKIN & HAIR
COUGHING
PO CHI (PHYSICAL ENERGY)
BLOOD
DRYNESS
HARVEST
STUBBORNNESS
MONEY
SENTIMENTALITY
RECTITUDE

WOOD

LIVER, GALLBLADDER
SOUR
SIGHT-EYES
GREEN
ANGER
SHOUTING
MUSCLES & TENDONS
TWITCHING
HUN CHI (PSYCHIC ENERGY)
SALIVA
WIND
BIRTH
HOSTILITY
COMPETITION
RATIONALITY
BENEVOLENCE

EARTH

STOMACH, SPLEEEN/PANCREAS
SWEET
TOUCH-SKIN
YELLOW
REMINISCENCE
SINGING
FLESH
HICCUPING
YUAN CHI (PRIMAL ENERGY)
VITAL ESSENCE
HUMIDITY
MATURITY
AMBITION
MIND
TRANQUILITY
TRUSTFULNESS

WATER

BLADDER, KIDNEYS
SALTY
HEARING-EARS
BLACK
FEAR
GROANING
BONE
SHIVERING
CHING CHI (CREATIVE ENERGY)
SEXUAL ESSENCE
COLD
STORAGE
DESIRE
ALCOHOL
DESIRE
WISDOM

eyes, headache, etc. we would want to strengthen or tonify the Metal element (lungs) to control the Wood. The creative and control cycles occur as natural phenomena. However, when any one of the elements is either too strong or too weak, disharmony results. Keep in mind as you use the five elements theory that there are always exceptions to the rule.

Your Body – The Greatest Healer

Americans are a perfect example of an overfed and undernourished country. We are constantly bombarded by information on nutrition from food companies, current faddists, and diet cultists, yet the picture is very incomplete. According to the Chinese point of view, the body is looked at as a whole, working together in harmony. Just as every little screw and bolt on a machine has an important purpose, if one part is broken the whole suffers. Our body is a very intricate machine that works together as a whole. Western medicine tends to focus on only the diseased part of the body. Then it tries to attack and kill the diseased cells, not taking into account why those cells are diseased to begin with. It is not because the cells are exposed to viruses and bacteria. We are constantly exposed to these; our mouth is full of bacteria. Yet why is it that some people break down and get sick and others do not, when both are exposed to the same pathogens?

Our body is equipped with a healing mechanism that is greater than any invention. It is so unique that it has this system that can repair the body's disharmonies, given the right chance to do so. Through inappropriate lifestyle, diet, thoughts, and actions, we abuse the workings of this delicate system. Always keep in mind that

12

the body's own healing system is very powerful. Suppressing a headache with aspirin does not take away the underlying cause. The headache is a warning of some disharmony. Thus, we should work on the underlying cause and use natural healing methods to enhance the immune system so the body can heal itself.

We seek to help the body to heal, not interfere with it. Often our surroundings do not give us the proper chance to heal ourselves, beginning with the bombardment of chemicals into our soil, food, water, and life, in general. These chemicals can accumulate in the liver and become very toxic. Another significant chemical pollution occurs in meats. Meat animals are routinely injected with steroids (female hormones) to fatten them quickly and antibiotics to control rampant diseases. These drug residues remain in the meat. The steroids in turn are causing men to become more feminine and have problems with impotency and sterility, and women to experience premature aging and general disharmonies in their endocrine systems and menstrual cycles.

Chinese View of the Body

The Chinese view the being as an intricate whole made up of these essential components: energy (also called chi or qi), blood, body fluids, jing, and shen (spirit). If any one of these components is missing, you cannot have life. Energy comes in many forms with many different actions. In general, chi is like life force. Energy cannot be destroyed, only transformed. The body is a network of pathways filled with energy; these are called meridians. In a healthy person this life force or energy flows evenly along these channels. When the energy becomes blocked, disease results. Acupunc-

13

ture can be of great value to facilitate the flow of energy through these pathways.

Chi (the yang component) is closely related to blood (the yin component). Blood supplies the nutritive aspect in the body and nourishes chi. Movement of blood is dependent upon the energy.

Body fluids are of two types: jin are the thin, refined fluids such as sweat, tears, and tissue fluids and ye are the thick, lubricating fluids such as spinal fluid and synovial (joint) fluids.

Jing is the "essence of life" found in the egg, sperm, marrow, and brain ("the sea of marrow") and stored in the kidneys. At the time of conception, the fetus absorbs this vital essence from the egg and the sperm. All of our chromosomes at that time give us our jing. Thus, we are born with a certain amount. Then throughout our lives we use up our jing until we die. The fast-paced American lifestyle uses up jing at a very rapid rate. For this reason women here go through an early menopause and cannot safely bear children for as many years as in more natural cultures. Spiritual cultivation is very important for the proper development of our vital essence.

The shen or spirit gives us intuition, instincts, and the ability to comprehend. Shen is stored in the heart.

Organs of the Body

The Chinese view the body organs as couples consisting of a yin organ and a yang organ. Each pair also is corresponded to one of the five elements.

Corresponding to Fire are the heart and small intestines. The heart houses the spirit, governs blood, externally manifests in the tongue, has taste as its sensory function, and joy as its related emotion. The small intestines absorb fluids and as one of the hollow organs are responsible for the transporting of excretions.

Also related to the Fire element are the triple heater and the pericardium which are functions rather than organs. The triple heater is responsible for communication between the three cavities in the trunk and helps with fluid metabolism in the body. The pericardium surrounds and protects the heart.

Corresponding to the element of Earth is the pair, spleen and stomach. The spleen transforms and transports food into usable food essence (the waste is transported to the intestines), produces blood, opens to the mouth, controls muscles, and is responsible for keeping the blood in the vessels (thus, bruising easily is a sign of weak spleen function). The related emotion is worry (excessive thinking). Reference made to the spleen in the Chinese system also includes the pancreas organ, since they function together. The stomach breaks down and "ripens" the food and transports it downward.

The pair corresponding to the Metal element is the lungs and large intestines. The main functions of the lungs are breathing, regulating water metabolism, and to disperse and descend the chi throughout the body; lungs open out to the nose, and control the skin, pores, and skin hair. Sadness is the related emotion. The large intestines excrete wastes from the body and absorb water.

15

The pair related to the Wood element is the liver and gall bladder. The liver houses the soul, controls tendons, is responsible for keeping the energy flowing (thus, when the energy is obstructed, look to the liver), stores blood, and manifests externally in the eyes. Anger is the emotion of the liver. The gall bladder stores and excretes bile, protects the nervous system from overreaction, and helps to normalize a person emotionally.

Related to the Water element are the kidneys and urinary bladder. The kidneys store jing, are responsible for growth, development, and reproduction, produce marrow, form brain and spinal cord, control bones, open to the ears, and balance body fluid metabolism. The related emotion is fear. The urinary bladder stores and excretes urine.

Causes of Disease

Just below the surface of the skin lies a layer of energy that acts as a protective shield. In a healthy person this shield is strong and without gaps, as a barrier of protection should be: impervious to external factors. If, however, there are weak spots in this shield and external factors can penetrate into the body, we have disease. This is roughly equivalent to the immune system. If one's immune system is strong, one does not "catch the bug." For example, some people have the A.I.D.S. virus and show no symptoms of it; others catch it and die within weeks. That is the difference between strong protective chi and chi that is weak and vulnerable to attack from the outside. In the Chinese perception of disease, this would be one category of the causes of disease, namely, external factors. These external factors include the following environmental conditions: cold, heat, summer heat, dryness, dampness, and wind.

Diseases can also arise as a result of internal factors. These include the following emotions: joy, grief, anger, depression, worry, melancholy, and fear. These reflect the mental state induced by one's environment. That in itself does not cause disease. However, when emotions are very intense or long lasting, disharmony or disease can result. Mental attitude is very important for good health. By calming one's mind many physical problems disappear.

An interesting survey done in China on a group of cancer patients showed that 95% had been physically or mentally tortured during the Cultural Revolution (1965-1975). During that harsh period intellectuals were tortured and even husbands and wives betrayed each other for the sake of the Party. You could not trust anyone with your innermost feelings and thoughts. These people built up frustration, depression, and anger; these destructive emotions in turn became cancers. So remember the importance of emotional balance in maintaining good health.

We must have a channel to release any excessive emotion, be it exercises such as a T'ai Chi Ch'uan or Chi Gong, breathing techniques, acupuncture, etc. These activities can help to regulate emotions.

Other miscellaneous causes of disease would include traumatic injury, stagnant blood or mucus, improper exercise, improper activities, and improper diet. Traumatic injuries would include accidents, incisions, sprains, burns, and animal or insect bites. Stagnancy of the blood and mucus cause blocks in the energy pathways; a good example is tumors. Either too much or too little exercise can cause disease. Improper activities would include too much sex, overworking, and overexertion. Excessive sex is particularly injurious to the kidneys, the storehouse of our jing. Improper diet could be eating too little for proper nourishment of the body, overeating, or eating too much of the wrong foods, such as too much raw, cold, greasy, or spicy foods.

Overeating is a very common imbalance in this country that causes many diseases. Americans constantly overeat because they do not know how to eat and tend to eat very fast. By slowly chewing one's food properly, the body will tell you when to stop. Also, people reach out to food and use it as an escape. Eating in a relaxed frame of mind is essential to good digestion and assimilation of nutrients.

It has been found in animal experiments that if one group is allowed to eat as much as desired and another group is starved every second day, the first group has five times more tendency toward spontaneous cancer. An interesting statistic: U.S. leads the world in both protein consumption per person and the incidence of cancer. Protein is needed, but an excessive amount causes problems. Meat companies have led us to believe that we need far more protein than is really healthy. Moderation is essential to good health.

What do we do after the disease comes? The Western approach is to kill the bacteria and suppress the symptoms, thus driving the disease deeper into the body. The Chinese way supports the body and lets it do the killing of the bacteria. Supporting the body with tonification reinforces the body's healing energy. Remember that the body can heal itself if given the proper chance. We may need to give it a little help through nutritional measures or herbal medicines.

Fasting or light eating is sometimes recommended during an illness, such as a cold, so as not to detract from the body's healing by having to digest heavy foods. Thus, the body can draw on its resources at such times if needed. Antibiotics, on the other hand, weaken the immune system, make one more prone to illness, cause the immune system to become lazy, and generally interfere with the natural healing process.

There are many possible supportive measures through food and herbs that can be taken. In many instances, along with supporting the body we also need to concurrently detoxify or sedate it. This is the Chinese approach to disease. For cancer patients in some hospitals in China, doctors combine the killing aspects of chemotherapy and radiation with the supportive measures of traditional Chinese medicine, including proper diet, herbs, Chi Gong exercises and acupuncture. This has produced a longer life expectancy than the conventional killing approach alone. Then some hospitals treat cancer patients solely with Chinese medicine; this group shows the longest life expectancy with many total remissions.

The Eight Differentiations

In order to more clearly understand the energy of the patient and the nature and location of the disease, the Chinese have developed these principles. Internal and external serves to locate the area of disease. Internal diseases are treated differently than external ones. Deficient and excess determine the relative strength of the patient or the disease. Cold and hot give indications of the nature of the individual or the pathogens. Yin and yang give the overall picture of the condition. Together these eight differenti-

19

ations can provide a fairly accurate picture of both the individual being treated and the disease at hand. Often there is a mixture of symptoms, not a clear cut condition. These principles provide a basis to better understand the seemingly contradictive symptoms.

Prevention

As we increase our awareness of health, we can hopefully maintain a state of balance within the body, and become more responsible for our health. Too often we suffer from our inappropriate actions and thoughts. Chinese nutrition stresses the prevention of disease. In <u>The Yellow Emperor's Classic of Internal Medicine</u>, written 2000-3000 years ago, it was said that, "A doctor who treats a disease after it has happened is a mediocre doctor, but a doctor who treats a disease before it happens is a superior doctor." We as individuals can choose to be one kind of doctor or the other.

Prevention of disease includes proper nutrition, emotional balance, proper exercise, as well as nourishing our spirit. As we nourish body, mind, and spirit we maintain a state of balance. Preventative maintenance is the most sensible route to take. As The Yellow Emperor states: "The sages of ancient times emphasized not the treatment of disease, but rather the prevention of its occurrence. To administer medicine to disease which has already developed and to suppress revolts which have already begun is comparable to the behavior of one who begins to dig a well after he has become thirsty or one who begins to forge weapons after he has engaged in battle. Would these actions not be too late?"

20

Guidelines for a Balanced Diet

As every body is unique, there will always be variations according to individual needs. A few basic guidelines, however, are appropriate as we seek a way of eating that creates balance and harmony. Frame of mind is of utmost importance at mealtime; relax and slowly chew your food for optimal digestion and assimilation. The dinner table is not the place to discuss the day's problems. Chewing is a major part of digestion. Remember, your stomach does not have teeth. Digestion, particularly of the starches, begins in the mouth. Foods that are difficult to thoroughly masticate, such as sesame seeds, should be ground before eating.

The best ways of preparing foods are steaming, stir frying in water, stewing (boiling, as in soups), or baking. Even the best quality oils become hard to digest when heated. So, if oil is desired, put it on after the food is cooked. Foods should be eaten in their wholeness, when possible. Only peel fruits or vegetables if the peel is hard to digest or contaminated with chemical sprays. Search out organically grown foods to avoid the toxic chemical residues of commercial growing processes. To clean foods thoroughly one may wash them in salt water. Also avoid irradiated foods and microwave ovens.

The best utensils for cooking in are glass, earthenware, or stainless steel. One should avoid cooking in aluminum or copper; these metals can easily leach into the food.

One's diet should follow the seasons, eating what grows locally. Nature has the perfect plan in providing the appropriate foods for the given season. The fruits and vegetables that ripen in

21

the summertime tend to be on the cooling side, because their growth period occurs during the cooler months. In wintertime we will tend toward a more warming diet. Also, one should eat a wide variety of foods for good balance.

Most vegetables should be at least lightly cooked as raw vegetables tend to be difficult to digest. Foods should never be eaten cold because cold foods put out the digestive fire, so to say. This is particularly upsetting to the female menstrual cycle as the stomach sits right beside the liver which is responsible for storing blood. Cooling off the stomach can lead to a stagnant blood condition and a difficult menstrual period. Frozen foods, such as ice cream, are a very unhealthy item, as well as iced drinks. Neither should we consume foods that are so hot that they burn the mouth or stomach.

Overeating is a serious problem in America that leads to many health problems. It is best to stop eating before the "full" point. Also, eating just before retiring is not healthy. One should take the last meal at least 3 hours before going to bed. This will not only result in better digestion, but also a more restful sleep. Late eating also tends to easily be stored as unwanted pounds. One should wake up with a good appetite for breakfast. This is the meal that provides us with the fuel or energy for much of the day, so make this a very nutritious meal.

It is best not to consume an excessive amount of fluids before, during, or after meals as this tends to dilute digestive juices and weaken digestive function. Nuts and seeds contain a large proportion of oil and should be eaten as fresh as possible. Because most people do not chew nuts

22

well, grinding them into powder makes them more easily digested. Beans should be soaked prior to cooking for at least a few hours; always discard the soak water and cook them in fresh water. For a person with particularly weak digestion it is best to cook grains "soupy", with additional water and cooking time. Always avoid highly processed foods and keep meals as simple as possible.

The following proportions would be an appropriate and well balanced diet for a reasonably healthy person (certain disharmonies may necessitate variations):

Vegetarian: 2/5 grains
2/5 vegetables and fruits
1/5 nuts and legumes

Lacto–Ovo–
Vegetarian: 2/5 grains
2/5 vegetables and fruits
1/5 eggs and dairy products (and nuts and legumes as a minor portion)

Meat eater: 4/10 grains
4/10 vegetables and fruits
1/10 meats
1/10 nuts and legumes

In all cases, a variety of grains should be consumed which may include such grains as brown rice, buckwheat, oats, millet, barley, corn, and wheat. Meats and eggs should be produced naturally, free of antibiotics and steroids, and not chemically preserved or processed.

SECTION

Foods

VEGETABLES

ALFALFA SPROUT

Nature: cooling
Actions: benefits spleen and stomach, dispels dampness, lubricates intestines
Conditions: swelling, constipation, skin lesions
Folk Remedies:
1. Swelling - boil tea and drink 3 times daily.
2. Constipation - eat raw alfalfa sprouts.
3. Skin lesions - apply mashed alfalfa sprouts; change poultice 3-4 times daily.

ASPARAGUS

Nature: cooling
Actions: clears heat, detoxifies, promotes blood circulation
Conditions: constipation, cancer, hypertension, high blood cholesterol, arteriosclerosis
Folk Remedies:
1. High cholesterol, hypertension, and arteriosclerosis - drink 1 glass daily of blender-made asparagus juice, including the pulp; add 1 teaspoon of honey.
2. Breast cancer - boil asparagus with dandelions; drink the liquid and apply the poultice to the area.
3. Constipation - eat asparagus with cabbage, lightly steamed.

BAMBOO SHOOT

Nature: cooling
Actions: strengthens the stomach, relieves food retention, resolves mucus, promotes diureses, cuts or emulsifies grease, relieves alcohol intoxication
Conditions: diabetes, indigestion, stomach distention and fullness due to greasy food, diarrhea, dysentery, rectal prolapse, edema
Contraindications: Not to be used after giving birth as they may trigger the cleansing of an old illness, manifesting in skin lesions.

Folk Remedies:

1. <u>Diarrhea, dysentery, and rectal prolapse</u> – cook bamboo shoots with rice.
2. <u>Swelling due to kidney, heart, or liver disease</u> – drink tea of bamboo shoots and winter melon rind.
3. <u>Diabetes</u> – blend bamboo shoots and celery juice, warm up and drink 1 cup twice daily. Eat plenty of bamboo shoots.
4. <u>Stomach distention and fullness</u> – make tea from bamboo shoots, ginger, and orange peel, and drink.

BEET

Nature: cooling
Actions: nourishes blood, tonifies the heart, calms the spirit, lubricates the intestines, cleanses the liver
Conditions: anemia, heart weakness, irritability, restlessness, habitual constipation, herpes, constipation, liver intoxica-

tion, i.e., from drugs

Contraindications: Not for someone with a history
of kidney stones because of the
oxalic acid content.

Folk Remedies:
1. Constipation - make beet soup, or combine beets
   with cabbage.
2. Blood deficiency - cook beets with black beans
   and peanuts.
3. Liver cleansing - drink beet top tea, or
   combine with dandelions and make tea.
4. Herpes - do a 3 day fast with vegetable broth*
   and beet top tea.

*Basic vegetable broth for detoxification can
be made by simmering carrots and carrot tops,
celery, dandelions, asparagus, and squash.

BELL PEPPER

Nature: slightly warming
Actions: strengthens stomach, improves appetite,
promotes blood circulation, removes
stagnant food, reduces swelling
Conditions: indigestion, decreased appetite,
swelling, frostbite, food retention
Folk Remedies:
1. Indigestion and food retention - make green
   pepper tea.
2. Frostbite - wash affected area in bell pepper
   and cinnamon tea, and drink the tea.
3. Decreased appetite and anorexia - mix bell
   pepper with black pepper and dry fry (no oil).
   Or lightly fry chunks of bell pepper with oil.

BOK CHOY

Nature: cooling
Actions: clears heat, lubricates the intestines, removes stagnant food, quenches thirst, promotes digestion
Conditions: food retention, constipation, indigestion, diabetes
Folk Remedies:
1. Food retention – boil tea or soup from bok choy and orange peel.
2. Indigestion – eat pickled bok choy.
3. Constipation – cook bok choy with beets.
4. Thirst – drink bok choy and cucumber juice.

BROCCOLI

Nature: cooling
Actions: clears heat, promotes diuresis, brightens eyes, clears summer heat problems. This vegetable is weak in action.
Conditions: conjunctivitis, nearsightedness, difficult urination, irritability
Folk Remedies:
1. Clear heat – eat lightly steamed broccoli.
2. Conjunctivitis – drink carrot and broccoli tea.
3. Urinary difficulty – combine broccoli with Chinese cabbage and make soup.

BURDOCK ROOT (GOBO)

Nature: cooling
Actions: clears heat, dispels wind, brightens vision
Conditions: common cold of the wind-heat type, sore

throat, measles, conjunctivitis, mumps
Contraindications: Not to be used in cases of diarrhea.
Folk Remedies:
1. Conjunctivitis - boil tea and expose eyes to the steam then drink the tea.
2. Common cold and measles - drink burdock tea and sweat.
3. Mumps - make burdock and dandelion tea, apply locally and drink the tea.

CABBAGE (RED OR GREEN)

Nature: cooling
Actions: clears heat, lubricates intestines, stops cough
Conditions: constipation, whooping cough, hot flashes, common colds, frostbite
Folk Remedies:
1. Common cold - take 1/4 head cabbage and 3 green onions, boil 10 minutes and drink the liquid, and sweat.
2. Whooping cough - make cabbage tea and add 2 teaspoons honey to lubricate the lungs (or add apricot kernel).
3. Frostbite - wash the area in warm cabbage and green onion tea.

CARROT

Nature: cooling
Actions: clears heat, detoxifies, strengthens all organs, benefits the eyes, relieves measles, lubricates the intestines

31

Folk Remedies:
1. <u>Night blindness</u> – drink lukewarm carrot juice.
2. <u>Diphtheria with sore throat</u> – drink carrot top tea.
3. <u>Indigestion</u> – make carrot tea and add a teaspoon of brown sugar or maltose.
4. <u>Measles</u> – make tea from carrots, water chestnut, and cilantro to induce eruption. It goes away after completely erupting.
5. <u>Skin lesions or eye weakness</u> – make tea or juice from carrots and carrot tops.
6. <u>Cancer</u> – to prevent, cook 1/2 stick carrot with Chinese black mushrooms and consume daily. Also drink carrot top tea.

CAULIFLOWER

Nature: cooling
Actions: lubricates the intestines, strengthens spleen. This vegetable is weak in action.
Conditions: constipation, weak digestion
Folk Remedies:
1. <u>Weak digestion</u> – eat lightly steamed cauliflower with bell pepper and celery.
2. <u>Constipation</u> – eat raw cauliflower in salad.

CELERY

Nature: cooling
Actions: tonifies kidney, stops bleeding, strengthens spleen and stomach, clears heat, lowers blood pressure, promotes diuresis
Folk Remedies:
1. <u>High Blood Pressure</u> (hypertension) – eat celery regularly; drink 3 cups lightly boiled celery

juice daily. Or drink lukewarm celery juice on an empty stomach daily.
2. Diabetes - drink 3 cups lightly boiled celery juice daily. Or combine celery, yam and pumpkin to make vegetable pie.
3. Whooping Cough - lightly steam celery juice, add a pinch of salt, take a warm glassful at 5 A.M. and at 7 P.M., three days in a row.
4. Insomnia - take celery and beet tops tea in the evening, 2 hours prior to bed time.

CHINESE CABBAGE (NAPA CABBAGE)

Nature: cold
Actions: clears heat, lubricates intestines, promotes urination
Conditions: irritability, restlessness, constipation, difficulty urinating
Folk Remedies:
1. Constipation or difficulty urinating - make Chinese cabbage soup.
2. Common cold (wind-cold type) - mix Chinese cabbage and ginger, simmer into tea, and sweat.

CHINESE CHIVE

Nature: warming
Actions: tonifies kidneys and sexual functions, removes dampness, warms up coldness
Conditions: cold stomachache, leukorrhea, diarrhea, bed-wetting, wet dreams, absences of menstrual period
Folk Remedies:
1. For the above conditions, boil Chinese chive tea for 25-30 minutes.

2. Weak sexual functions – cook Chinese chives with black beans, black sesames, walnuts, sour plums, and 2 tsp. honey. Make into a paste and take 1 Tbsp. 3 times daily.

CILANTRO (CHINESE PARSLEY)

Nature: cooling
Actions: promotes sweating, strengthens digestion, promotes chi flow
Conditions: measles, common cold, indigestion, lack of appetite, chest and stomach fullness
Folk Remedies:
1. Measles – drink cilantro and mint tea to induce eruptions.
2. Common cold of the wind cold type – drink cilantro and ginger tea.
3. Common cold of the wind heat type – drink cilantro and mint tea.
4. Qi stagnation – drink cilantro and orange peel tea.

CORN

Nature: cooling
Actions: stops bleeding, promotes diureses, strengthens gall bladder, lowers blood pressure, clears heat, detoxifies
Conditions: difficult urination, gallstones, hepatitis, jaundice, hypertension
Folk Remedies:
1. Hypertension, jaundice, and gallstones – eat corn regularly and drink fresh cornsilk tea.
2. Detoxify and clear heat – drink cornsilk and dandelion tea.

34

3. Swelling or difficulty urinating - drink cornsilk and pearl barley tea.
4. High blood pressure - drink cornsilk and chrysanthemum tea.
5. Bloody urine - drink corn and lotus root tea.

CUCUMBER

Nature: cooling
Actions: clears heat, quenches thirst, relieves irritability, promotes diuresis
Conditions: swelling of the extremities, jaundice, diarrhea, epilepsy
Contraindications: Eating cucumbers to excess will cause dampness.
Folk Remedies:
1. Swelling of the extremities and jaundice - boil tea from cucumber skins.
2. Diarrhea - use 2 teaspoons of dried cucumber meal mixed with rice porridge.
3. Epilepsy - boil tea from cucumber vines.
4. Hot, scratchy, or swollen (puffy) eyes - apply grated cucumber packs to closed eyes; leave on 20 minutes.

DAIKON RADISH (WHITE CARROT)

Nature: cooling
Actions: removes stagnant food, moistens lungs, resolves mucus, quenches thirst, relieves alcohol intoxication
Conditions: bronchitis, sore throat, dry cough, coughing of blood, painful urination, excess of mucus, alcohol intoxication, food retention

Folk Remedies:

1. <u>Bronchitis or sore throat</u> – make daikon juice and add 2 drops of ginger juice; drink 1 cup lukewarm, 3 times daily.
2. <u>Dry cough with yellow sputum</u> – take warm daikon and water chestnut juice with 1 tsp. honey.
3. <u>Burns</u> – apply grated daikon alone or mixed with aloe vera gel.
4. <u>Alcohol intoxication</u> – drink daikon juice before and after the alcohol.

DANDELION

Nature: cooling
Actions: clears heat, detoxifies, anti-tumor
Conditions: toxic skin lesions, bug bites, poison oak blisters, conjunctivitis, liver heat rising, beginning stages of common cold

Folk Remedies:

1. <u>Toxic skin lesions</u> – apply crushed, fresh leaves; change poultice hourly.
2. <u>Conjunctivitis (liver heat rising)</u> – make tea or juice.
3. <u>Common cold</u> – make tea from fresh dandelions (the whole plant), mint, and licorice.
4. <u>Breast lumps and tumors</u> – apply dandelion and ginger poultices.

Note: Dandelion has been found to be extremely effective in inhibiting bacteria, virus, and fungus. It is considered to be a natural anti-biotic, similar in action to goldenseal root (Hydrastis canadensis).

EGGPLANT

Nature: cooling
Actions: relieves pain, promotes diureses, reduces swelling, removes blood stagnation
Conditions: abdominal pain, dysentery, hot diarrhea, painful urination, frostbite, canker sores, snake and scorpion bites
Contraindications: Not to be used for cold type problems.
Folk Remedies:
1. Bites – apply fresh to absorb toxins.
2. Jaundice and hepatitis – eat eggplant and rice 3 times daily for 1 week.
3. Swelling and edema – dry the eggplant and grind to a meal; take 1 teaspoon in warm water 3 times daily.
4. Frostbite – soak area in eggplant tea.
5. Canker sores – charcoal eggplant and apply locally.

GARLIC

Nature: hot
Actions: anti-viral, anti-fungal, detoxifies meat and seafood, kills worms, removes stagnant food and stagnant blood, reduces abscess
Conditions: cancer and high blood cholesterol, infections, diarrhea, dysentery, vomiting, and coughing of blood
Contraindications: Not to be used with eye disorders.
Folk Remedies:
1. Vaginal infections – boil a bulb of garlic, cool to lukewarm, then douche with the liquid.

2. Coughing or vomiting of blood - apply crushed, peeled, raw garlic to the soles of both feet at the depression behind the ball of the foot, also known as "rushing spring" point; change the poultice every 4 hours.
3. Dysentery - mash 3-5 cloves of raw garlic, mix with warm water; drink every 2 hours.
4. Vomiting - cook together a bulb of garlic and 3 slices ginger; mix with a teaspoon of honey and some water.
5. Antidote for crab poisoning - cook garlic with crabs or other sea foods.
6. Earache or ear infection- put a few drops of garlic oil or juice in ear several times daily.
7. Intestinal worms - eat cooked garlic on an empty stomach; resume eating 3 hours later.

GREEN BEAN

Nature: warming
Actions: warms spleen and stomach, descends chi, tonifies kidneys, benefits chi
Conditions: burping, chest fullness and discomfort, whooping cough, hernia in children, chronic diarrhea, back pain due to kidney weakness
Folk Remedies:
1. Whooping cough - boil 1/2 cup green beans and 6 grams licorice in 1 1/2 cups water; boil down to 1 cup and add 2 of teaspoons honey. Drink the liquid.
2. Chronic diarrhea - steam green beans with rice.
3. Hernia in children - Dry fry green beans with fennel and then ground into powder. Take 1/2 tsp. each time, 3 times daily with lukewarm water. Also can be applied as a paste (green beans and fennel) to the navel with black

pepper.
4. Back pain — make soup with green beans, black beans, and azuki beans and a pinch of cinnamon powder.

KALE

Nature: warming
Actions: strengthens stomach, stops pains, promotes regrowth of tissue
Conditions: stomach or duodenal ulcers
Folk Remedies:
1. Ulcers — take 1/2 glass warm kale juice before each meal.

LETTUCE

Nature: neutral
Actions: invigorates chi, removes stagnation, reduces swelling, softens hardening. This vegetable is mild in action.
Conditions: skin lesions, abdominal pain, breast abscess, postpartum abdominal pain due to blood stagnation
Folk Remedies:
1. Skin lesions i.e. erysipelas — apply mashed lettuce, changing poultice 3 times daily and drink 1 cup of lukewarm lettuce juice, 3 times daily.
2. Breast abscess — make poultice and juice with dandelions. Drink the juice and apply with gauze pad externally.

LOTUS ROOT

Nature: cooling
Actions: very healing, clears heat, quenches thirst, relieves irritability, stops bleeding, strengthens the stomach, promotes diuresis, cools the blood
Conditions: difficult urination, vomiting blood, nosebleed, blood in stool or urine, hypertension, gastritis, colitis
Folk Remedies:
1. <u>Nosebleed and hypertension</u> – drink lotus root juice daily.
2. <u>Gastritis and colitis</u> – drink diluted lotus root juice.
3. <u>Vomiting or defecating blood</u> – cook 1/2 c. of lotus root starch with 1/2 c. of rice porridge until jelly like consistency; consume while lukewarm.
4. <u>Blood in the urine</u> – make tea of lotus root and bamboo leaves.

LOTUS SEED

Nature: neutral
Actions: strengthens kidneys, astringent, nutritive tonic
Conditions: kidney weakness, frequent urination, seminal emission, diarrhea
Folk Remedies:
1. <u>Nutritive tonic</u> – A delicious winter tonic soup can be made by boiling together lotus seeds, azuki (red) beans, and pearl barley and adding a dash of honey.
2. <u>Frequent urination, seminal emission, and diarrhea</u> – cook lotus seed with chunks of yam in rice porridge.

40

MUSHROOMS (BUTTON)

Nature: slightly cooling
Actions: induces measle eruptions, detoxifies, improves appetite, stops diarrhea, resolves phlegm, anti-tumor
Conditions: infectious hepatitis, measles, diarrhea, cough with copious mucus, low appetite
Folk Remedies:
1. Infectious hepatitis, leukocytopenia - take button mushrooms in the diet or in tea.
2. Measles - boil tea from button mushrooms and drink one cup 3 times daily. Or, cook with poi and drink the broth.

MUSHROOM (CHINESE BLACK OR SHITAKE)

Nature: neutral
Actions: strengthens stomach, promotes healing, lowers blood pressure, anti-tumor
Conditions: tumor, diabetes, hypertension, slow healing
Folk Remedies:
1. Tumors - boil tea from black mushrooms and drink 3 times daily, continuously. This can also be used as a preventative to stomach and cervical cancer. Used post surgery, this remedy can prevent metastasis (spreading) of the tumor cells. (The strongest anti-tumor mushroom is the Ganoderma or Ling Zhi variety.)
2. To clean toxins in the intestines - soak some Chinese black mushrooms, blend with the soak water; heat like soup and take on an empty stomach. One can also add a little ginger.

41

MUSHROOM (WHITE)

Nature: cold
Actions: clears summer heat, lowers blood pressure,
    anti-tumor, detoxifies
Conditions: hypertension, summer irritability and
    other summer heat problems, tumors
Contraindications: White mushrooms should not be
            used by those with skin problems
            or allergies or cold stomach.
Folk Remedies:
1. High blood cholesterol or hypertension - use
   common white mushrooms and cornsilk, and make
   soup or tea regularly.
2. Tumors - make mushroom soup or tea daily and
   drink 3 cups daily.
3. Summer heat problems - eat raw mushrooms in
   salad.

MUSTARD GREEN

Nature: warm
Actions: relieves common colds, promotes diureses,
        dissolves mucus, strengthens and lubri-
        cates intestines, ventilates lungs,
        increases appetite
Conditions: difficulty urinating, coughing of
        blood, dysentery, sore throat, loss of
        voice, copious white sputum
Folk Remedies:
1. Difficulty urinating - make tea from fresh
   mustard and drink frequently.
2. Coughing of blood - make raw mustard greens
   juice, mix with some lukewarm water and gradually drink.
3. Dysentery - charcoal mustard plant roots and
   grind into meal. Mix 6 ounces of meal with water

and add 1 teaspoon of honey; drink 2 times
daily.
4. Common cold (wind cold type) - drink tea of
mustard greens, cilantro and green onions and
try to sweat.
5. Copious white sputum - drink mustard seed tea.

PARSLEY

Nature: slightly warming
Actions: promotes digestion, removes stagnant food,
regulates flow of chi, induces measle
eruption
Conditions: food retention, indigestion, stomach
and abdominal fullness, measles,
seafood or meat poisoning
Contraindications: Overconsumption of parsley is
not beneficial for the eyes.
Folk Remedies:
1. Breast abscess - make juice from 1/2 pound
parsley; divide into 3 portions to be taken with
warm wine.
2. Measles - make parsley tea; drink and mix the
tea with wine to be used as a wash, externally
to induce eruption.
3. Food retention, indigestion, and fullness -
make tea of parsley, hawthorn berries, daikon
radish, and orange peels.

PARSNIP

Nature: warming
Actions: promotes sweating, dispels wind and
dampness, relieves pain, stops bleeding
(when charred)

Conditions: common cold of the wind cold type, headache, muscle ache, dizziness, arthritis, tetanus

Folk Remedies:
1. <u>Common cold (wind-damp-cold type)</u> – make parsnip and ginger tea.
2. <u>Arthritis of the wind cold type</u> – combine parsnip, cinnamon, black pepper, and dry ginger to make tea, and drink. Externally apply either mashed, fresh jalepeno pepper or dry jalepeno mixed with some ginger tea. (Refer to section on arthritis for more information.)

POTATO

Nature: cooling

Actions: relieves ulcer pain, strengthens spleen, harmonizes stomach, tonifies chi, lubricates intestines, promotes diureses

Conditions: stomach and duodenal ulcers, constipation, eczema, skin lesions, swelling, small physical stature.

Contraindications: Do not eat sprouted or green potatoes.

Folk Remedies:
1. <u>Ulcer pain or constipation</u> – make raw potato juice in the blender, mix with a small amount of honey; take 2 tablespoons every morning on an empty stomach. Make fresh daily.
2. <u>Eczema or other damp, exuding sores</u> – apply raw grated potato locally with gauze, change every 3 hours.
3. <u>Genital eczema</u> – apply raw grated potato at night; change 6 times; repeat for 3 days.
4. <u>Swelling</u> – make tea of grated potato and cucumber.

PUMPKIN (AND WINTER SQUASH)

Nature: cooling
Actions: kills worms, dispels dampness, reduces fever, relieves pain, stabilizes hyperactive fetus, stops dysentery, benefits diabetes
Conditions: dysentery, diabetes, ulcerations of the lower extremities, eczema, stomachache, the feeling of "steaming bones"*, intestinal worms, antidote for opium

Folk Remedies:
1. Burns – apply fresh pumpkin alone locally or mixed with aloe vera gel.
2. Lower limb ulcerations – apply dried pumpkin meal.
3. Intestinal worms – take 1 teaspoon pumpkin seed meal 3 times daily on an empty stomach.
4. Childhood vomiting – make tea from the pumpkin stem and top "cap".
5. Breast cancer – charcoal the "cap" and grind to powder. Take 1 teaspoon of the powder in 1 shot of rice wine 2 times daily. (The alcohol is a useful agent for increasing circulation and removing stagnancy.) The tumor is considered to be some type of stagnancy (blood, chi, mucus, etc.).
6. Hyperactive fetus – take 1 teaspoon pumpkin ash in sweet rice gruel (congee or porridge).
7. Diabetes – eat a slice of pumpkin with every meal or bake pie with pumpkin, yam, and potato.

* The sensation of heat deep in the body as if "steam in the bones" is part of a condition of yin exhaustion in the body, along with insomnia, irritability, flushed cheeks, heat, especially severe in late afternoon or evenings, night sweats, thirst, feverish sensation in palms and soles.

45

SCALLION (GREEN ONION)

Nature: hot
Actions: expels external pathogens, dispels wind and cold, induces sweating, anti-viral, and anti-bacterial
Conditions: common cold, measles, abscesses, arthritis of the "cold type"
Contraindication: Not to be used for the "heat type" arthritis. Not to be used for heat stages of common cold, characterized by fever, extreme thirst, and yellow sputum.

Folk Remedies:
1. Common cold - make tea by lightly boiling scallions of 5 minutes. Basil and scallion tea is also good.
2. Measles - drink scallion tea and apply raw, mashed scallions to the navel to draw out the measles.
3. Abscesses - mix raw scallions with egg white and apply; change poultice every 4 hours.
4. Arthritis pain - make scallion tea and soak painful area; apply mashed, cooked scallions to painful area. Scallion and clove tea is also good to drink.

SEAWEED

Nature: cold
Actions: softens hardenings, clears heat, detoxifies, benefits the thyroid gland, alkalinizes the blood, neutralizes radioactive material, benefits the lymphatic system, promotes diuresis, provides many minerals
Conditions: swollen lymph glands, goiters, cough,

46

lung abscess with thick, yellow, odoriferous mucus, edema, beriberi, fibroid tumors, nodules, lumps, cancer

Folk Remedies:
1. <u>Goiter</u> – make soup from dried (preferably green) orange peel, carrots, and seaweed.
2. <u>Lymph tuberculosis</u> – incorporate seaweeds into the diet for at least 2 months.
3. <u>Cough and lung abscess</u> – powder seaweed and mix with honey; these can be rolled into pills.
4. <u>Lumps, nodules, and tumors</u> – make tea from seaweed, peach kernel and green orange peels to take internally. Externally, make poultice of seaweed, ginger, and dandelion and apply locally.

Note: There are many varieties of seaweed that can be easily incorporated into soups, stir fry dishes, etc. A delicious healthful appetizer can be made with hiziki or arame (looks like thin black noodles), a little soy sauce, honey, and rice vinegar.

SNOW PEA

Nature: cold
Actions: strengthens middle warmer, detoxifies, relieves vomiting, promotes diuresis, relieves belching, stops dysentery, aids lactation, quenches thirst
Conditions: chronic diarrhea, dysentery, difficulty urinating, lower abdominal distention and fullness, diabetes, lactostasis, vomiting
Folk Remedies:
1. <u>Diabetes</u> – cook snow peas, then blend juice; take 1/2 cup 2 times daily.

2. Hypertension – make juice from fresh snow peas; take 1/2 cup 2 times daily.
3. Diarrhea – cook snow peas in sweet rice and take it every meal until relieved.
4. Lactostasis – consume steamed snow peas frequently.

SOYBEAN SPROUT

Nature: cooling
Actions: promotes diuresis, clears heat
Conditions: food retention, stomach heat, swelling, arthritis, spasms
Folk Remedies:
1. Hypertension – boil tea for 4 hours; drink lukewarm, over a period of 1 month.
2. Warts – eat only steamed soybean sprouts for 3 days consecutively without anything else.

SPINACH

Nature: cooling
Actions: strengthens all organs, lubricates intestines, promotes urination, ventilates the chest, quenches thirst
Conditions: constipation, thirst, tightness in chest, inability to urinate, night blindness, alcohol intoxication, diabetes
Contraindications: Not to be used with diarrhea, or a history of kidney stones. Also, spinach does not mix well with tofu or dairy products due to the unhealthy combination

that results from the oxalic
acid in the spinach and the
calcium foods. This can lead to
crystallized stones in the
kidneys or elsewhere.

Folk Remedies:
1. Acute Conjunctivitis - simmer spinach and
   chrysanthemum flowers; drink the liquid.
2. Night blindness - fresh spinach juice, drink 1
   cup 2 times daily.
3. Diabetes - boil tea from spinach and chicken
   gizzard, drink 1 cup 3 times daily.
4. Constipation, urinary obstruction, headache -
   drink spinach soup.

SQUASH (SUMMER SQUASH, ZUCCHINI)

Nature: cooling
Actions: clears heat, detoxifies, promotes diuresis, quenches thirst, relieves fidgetiness
Conditions: skin lesions, difficulty urinating,
edema, summer heat, irritability,
thirst
Contraindications: Not to be used in beriberi
or scabies.
Folk Remedies:
1. Burns - preserve cut up squash until it becomes
   liquid (usually 6 - 12 months) and apply the
   liquid to the burn.
2. Edema in the extremities or the abdomen - cook
   squash with vinegar until soggy and eat on empty
   stomach or make tea from squash skin.
3. Summer heat and irritability - eat squash as a
   salad.
4. Jaundice - drink tea made from squash skin, 1
   cup 3 times daily.

SWEET POTATO (YAM)

Nature: cooling
Actions: strengthens spleen and stomach function, tonifies chi, clears heat, detoxifies, increases the production of milk
Conditions: bloody stools, diarrhea, constipation, jaundice, edema, ascites, night blindness, diabetes, breast abscess, boils, skin lesions
Contraindications: Overeating sweet potatoes will cause gas, heartburn, indigestion, abdominal distention and acid regurgitation.

Folk Remedies:

1. Night blindness - cook yam or sweet potato with animal liver (preferably goat).
2. Jaundice - cook yam soup with squash and pearl barley.
3. Shingles and breast abscess - apply grated, raw yam locally or mix in a pinch of borax.
4. Eczema (particularly genital eczema) - make tea with sweet potato and a pinch of salt and bathe the area. Sprinkle afterwards with some natural talcum powder.
5. Poison insect bites - mash yam or sweet potato with honey and apply.
6. Cirrhosis of the liver and accompanying edema in the abdomen - apply to the navel a mixture of mashed sweet potato and brown sugar; change hourly.
7. Diabetes - cook soup with winter melon.
8. Bloody stools - mix sweet potato powder or yam powder with honey.

TARO ROOT

Nature: neutral, although raw is slightly toxic
Actions: clears heat, reduces swelling, benefits spleen, regulates digestive system
Conditions: swollen lymph glands, nodules, goiters, externally for pain from tendonitis, sprains, traumas, snake bites, bee stings
Contraindications: If you eat too much, can cause food retention and stomach pains. Externally, can cause allergic reaction in some people. An antidote for this would be to apply fresh ginger juice. Also, do not eat taro root raw.

Folk Remedies:
1. Externally for infections such as pleurisy, peritonitis, appendicitis, joint pain, sciatica, back pain, arthritis - mix together peeled taro root and ginger, mixed into a paste with some flour and water, and apply to the affected area. Cover with a cloth. During the winter time, heat up the paste and apply. Change daily and always apply fresh.
2. Snake bite, bee sting, and bug bites - mash taro root with a pinch of salt and apply locally.
3. Blisters that contain fluid - charcoal taro to ash, mix with sesame oil and apply to blister.
4. Swollen lymph glands, nodules, scrofula, goiter, and T.B. - dry taro root, grind to powder, then take equal parts of water chestnuts and jelly fish and boil into tea. Take the liquid and mix with the taro root powder; roll into pills the size of mung beans, take 2 T. of pills 3 times daily with warm water.

51

TURNIP

Nature: cooling
Actions: clears heat, removes dampness, removes stagnant food, detoxifies, stops cough
Conditions: boils, breast abscesses, diabetes, tinea (ringworm), baldness in children
Folk Remedies:
1. Abscesses – apply grated raw turnip bulbs mixed with a tablespoon of salt.
2. Balding in children – charcoal turnip greens and mix with sesame oil; apply to bald spots.

WATERCRESS

Nature: cooling
Actions: clears heat, quenches thirst, lubricates lungs, promotes diuresis
Conditions: thirst, irritability, restlessness, sore and dry throat, cough with yellow sputum
Contraindications: Not to be used in diarrhea.
Folk Remedies:
1. Thirst, irritability, and sore throat – drink resh raw watercress juice.
2. Cough – boil tea from watercress and apricot kernels (or almonds). (It is best to remove the apex of the apricot kernel which is somewhat toxic.) Drink 1 cup 3 times daily.

WINTER MELON

Nature: cooling
Actions: clears heat, detoxifies, promotes urination, quenches thirst, relieves irritabil-

ity, dispels dampness, antidote for
seafood poisoning

Conditions: boils, skin lesions, ascites (edema in
the abdomen), difficult urination,
heatstroke

Folk Remedies:
1. Hives - make tea of winter melon skin and drink.
2. Chronic nephritis - cook winter melon with poi
and no salt.
3. Difficulty urinating - drink the fresh juice
with honey.
4. Heatstroke - make winter melon soup and drink 3
times daily.
5. Milk deficiency in nursing mother - cook winter
melon rind with trout.
6. Summer heat with continuous high fever - make
tea from winter melon rind and grapefruit seeds
(remove shells or crush seeds) and drink
constantly.

WINTER MELON SEED

Nature: cooling
Actions: promotes diuresis, resolves mucus, stops
cough, clears heat, detoxifies,
Conditions: coughing of blood, constipation,
intestinal abscess (appendicitis),
edema, leukorrhea

Folk Remedies:
1. Coughing of blood, constipation, and intestinal
abscess - make tea of the seeds.
2. Edema and leukorrhea - grind seeds into meal and
take 1 teaspoon with warm water 3 times daily.

APPLE

Nature: cooling
Actions: strengthens heart, tonifies chi, quenches thirst, promotes body fluids, lubricates lungs, resolves mucus
Conditions: dry throat, dehydration, indigestion, hypertension, constipation, chronic diarrhea
Folk Remedies:
1. Constipation – eat a fresh apple on an empty stomach.
2. Indigestion – eat an apple after each meal.
3. Diarrhea – take 2 teaspoons of powdered, dried apple 3 times daily on an empty stomach.
4. Cough with yellow sputum – drink apple juice.
5. Hypertension – eat 3 apples a day.
6. General cleansing – fast one day a week on apples, apple juice, and beet top tea. The apples contain pectin which acts as a broom in our intestines. For problems of a cold nature, heat the apples to decrease their cooling properties.

APRICOT

Nature: slightly cooling, slightly toxic if taken to excess
Actions: regenerates body fluids, clears heat, detoxifies, quenches thirst
Conditions: dehydration, thirst, cough
Contraindications: Too much injures bones and tendons and produces mucus; in children this can cause skin

rashes. Not good to eat during
pregnancy.

Folk Remedies:
1. <u>Summer thirst and dehydration</u> – eat fresh
apricots (no more than 5-10).
2. The inner kernel of the apricot seed is used to
ventilate lungs, descend rebellious chi,
lubricate intestines, relieve constipation,
relieve cough and asthma. One should remove the
apex of the kernel which is toxic.
3. <u>Cough</u> – make tea from ground apricot kernels,
adding a bit of honey.

BANANA

Nature: cold
Actions: clears heat, lubricates lungs, lubricates
intestines, lowers blood pressure, aids
alcohol intoxication
Conditions: constipation, thirst, cough, hemorrhoids, hypertension, alcohol intoxication
Contraindications: Not to be used in cold conditions.
Folk Remedies:
1. <u>Hemorrhoids and constipation</u> – eat a banana
every day on an empty stomach.
2. <u>Hypertension</u> – drink banana peel (organic) tea.
3. <u>Cough</u> – cook banana with a bit of sugar. Note,
this may not be appropriate for Americans who
already consume about 120 pounds of sugar a
year. If honey is substituted, do not cook
the honey.

CANTALOUPE

Nature: cold
Actions: clears heat, quenches thirst, relieves summer heat problems, eases urination
Conditions: summer heat thirst, lung abscess, irritability
Contraindications: Not for cold conditions, history of coughing or vomiting blood, diarrhea, ulcers, heart disease, or weak stomach. Melons rot easily in the stomach and thus should be eaten alone.
Folk Remedies:
1. To induce vomiting – take dried, ground cantaloupe seeds in warm water.

CHERRY

Nature: warming
Actions: benefits skin and overall body, rejuvenates, strengthens spleen, stimulates appetite, stops dysentery and diarrhea, quenches thirst, regenerates fluids, stops seminal emissions, prolongs life
Conditions: measles, burns, diarrhea, dysentery, thirst, premature ejaculation
Contraindications: Eaten in excess will cause nausea, vomiting, skin lesions and cause a person to feel hot. This injures the bones and tendons.
Folk Remedies:
1. Measles – drink fresh warmed cherry juice.
2. Burns – apply locally.
3. Enlarged thyroid or goiter – soak cherry pits in vinegar until they disintegrate, then apply

locally.
4. <u>Hernia pain</u> – fry cherry pits with vinegar, mash to powder; take 1 teaspoon per dose.

CHINESE DATE (RED OR BLACK JUJUBE)

Nature: neutral
Actions: strengthens spleen, tonifies yin, nourishes the body, tonifies blood, lubricates lungs, stops coughs, stops diarrhea, harmonizes within the body or within an herb formula (dates and licorice can reduce the harshness of a food or herb and unite the combination into action).
Conditions: yin deficiency, weak digestion, cough, night sweats, weakness, anemia, blood in urine, diarrhea, bruises
Contraindications: Too much creates mucus, distended stomach, and is hard on the teeth.
Folk Remedies:
1. <u>Blood in urine</u> – drink red date tea.
2. <u>Spontaneous sweating</u> – boil tea from 10 red dates and 10 preserved plums.

CHINESE PRUNE

These prunes are made from half ripened plums and have a sour flavor. They are more beneficial therapeutically than the sweet American variety that is made from fully ripened plums.
Nature: cooling
Actions: astringes intestines, stops diarrhea, kills worms, stops cough, consolidates the lungs, quenches thirst, promotes body

fluids. The sweet plums quench thirst, promote body fluids, and moisten the intestines.

Folk Remedies:
1. <u>Dysentery</u> – for both prevention (as before a trip to India or Mexico) and treatment, brew prune tea and take before meals on empty stomach.
2. <u>Intestinal worms</u> – make tea with prunes and black pepper.
3. <u>Fish bones stuck in the throat</u> – brew concentrated prune tea and add an equal part of rice vinegar; drink slowly. The herb clematis, powdered and mixed with rice vinegar could be given in an emergency, to dissolve a fish bone.
4. <u>Summer heat irritability</u> – drink prune juice.

COCONUT

Nature: warm
Actions: strengthens the body, reduces swelling, stops bleeding, kills worms, activates heart function
Conditions: weakness, nosebleeds, intestinal or skin worms
Folk Remedies:
1. <u>Worms</u> – every morning on an empty stomach, drink the juice and eat the meat of 1/2 coconut; wait 3 hours before eating anything else.
2. <u>Edema due to weak heart</u> – drink plenty of coconut juice.

FIG

Nature: cooling

Actions: clears heat, lubricates lungs and intestines, stops diarrhea

Conditions: dry cough, dry throat, lung heat, constipation, indigestion, hemorrhoids, prolapse of the rectum

Folk Remedies:

1. Lung heat symptoms – make tea from figs (preferably fresh).
2. Hemorrhoids – bathe area in fig tea.
3. Asthma – blend fig juice and drink 3 times daily.
4. Hernia – drink fig and fennel tea.

GRAPE

Nature: warming

Actions: very tonifying (particularly the red or purple varieties), nourishes blood, strengthens bones and tendons, tonifies chi, harmonizes stomach, promotes diuresis, relieves irritability

Conditions: cold type arthritis, tendonitis, painful urination, hepatitis, jaundice, anemia, flu

Contraindications: Not to be used in constipation. Grape wine should not be combined with fatty foods because it can result in phlegm and heat that rises to the heart and can cause strokes and heart attacks. Also, excessive consumption of grapes leads to constipation.

Folk Remedies:

1. Anemia – eat raisins.
2. Arthritis (cold type) and tendonitis – make grape vine tea and add some grape wine. The

moderate use of grape wine can be of benefit in cold environments and cold conditions.
3. Hepatitis and jaundice – make grape tea.
4. Flu – drink grape juice.

GRAPEFRUIT

Nature: cold
Actions: strengthens stomach, aids digestion, circulates chi, detoxifies alcohol intoxication
Conditions: decreased appetite, weak digestion, stomach fullness, alcohol intoxication, dry cough
Folk Remedies:
1. Dry cough – cook 4 grapefruit slices with either pork or cabbage.
2. Chronic cough – make tea from about 20 grapefruit seeds, adding a bit of honey; drink 3 times daily.
3. Grapefruit peel is warming and can be used to dispel cold, regulate chi, aid digestion, dry dampness, resolve sputum, aid wind-cold cough, stomach distention and scratchy throat. Make tea from the dried peel.
4. Jaundice and stomach distention – char and powder grapefruit peel; take a teaspoon with warm water 3 times daily.
5. Gastritis or inflammation of the stomach – make tea from aged grapefruit peel, green tea leaves, and 2 slices of fresh ginger; drink all day.
6. Frostbite – wash or soak area in grapefruit peel tea.

61

HAWTHORN BERRY

Nature: cooling
Actions: strengthens spleen, removes stagnant food, invigorates blood, dissolves sputum, relieves stagnant chi, aids digestion
Conditions: stuck food (especially for meat eaters), bloody stools, abdominal pain, absence of menstruation due to blood stagnation, poor appetite, hypertension, high cholesterol
Folk Remedies:
1. Child with no appetite - give the berries or tea daily.
2. Hypertension - drink tea daily.

LEMON

Nature: cooling
Actions: regenerates body fluids, harmonizes stomach, regulates chi, quenches thirst
Conditions: sore throat, dry mouth, stomach distention
Folk Remedies:
1. Hypertension - make tea from 1 peeled lemon, 10 fresh water chestnuts, and 2 1/2 cups of water; drink once daily.
2. Sore throat - drink lemon tea with honey.

LITCHI FRUIT

Nature: warm and astringent
Actions: nourishes blood, calms spirit, soothes liver, regulates chi

Conditions: hernia, weak and deficient conditions, irritability, restless heart
Contraindications: Over consumption can lead to nosebleed, feverish sensation, thirst, and can induce the onset of smallpox or chicken pox. Not to be used in any type of heat condition.

Folk Remedies:
1. Weak conditions, blood deficiency – take dried litchi and black jujube date and boil tea (7 of each); drink daily.
2. Bed-wetting – eat 10 dried litchis daily.
3. Nausea, vomiting, burping, and belching – take dried litchi with the kernel, charcoal, powder and take with warm water.
4. Bleeding after birth or abortion – take 7 dried litchis, mash and boil with 2 cups of water; reduce to 1 cup, drink 3 times daily until the bleeding stops.
5. Hernia – take litchi kernel, bake and grind to powder; take 1 teaspoon on an empty stomach daily. Or, grind the litchi kernel, mix with rice wine and take every morning on an empty stomach.

LOQUAT

Nature: neutral
Actions: lubricates dryness, stops cough, harmonizes stomach, descends rebellious chi, calms liver
Conditions: dry mouth, thirst, irritability, dry cough, nausea, vomiting
Folk Remedies:
1. Vomiting and nausea – boil tea.
2. Cough – eat fresh.

MANGO

Nature: neutral
Actions: regenerates body fluids, stops cough, stops thirst, strengthens stomach
Conditions: cough, thirst, poor digestion, enlarged prostate
Folk Remedies:
1. Enlarged prostate - boil mango peel and seed into tea.
2. Weak digestion - drink mango juice.

MULBERRY

Nature: slightly cold
Actions: quenches thirst, detoxifies, nourishes blood, tonifies kidneys, lubricates lungs, relieves constipation, calms the spirit, promotes diureses
Conditions: thirst, irritability, dry mouth, diabetes, anemia, constipation, back pain due to kidney weakness, alcohol intoxication, lymph node enlargement
Folk Remedies:
1. Cough - take 2 teaspoons 2 times daily of mulberry syrup, made by cooking mulberries on low flame until they dissolve, then adding honey and cooking down to a thick syrup.
2. Constipation - drink mulberry juice.
3. Insomnia - boil mulberry tea and take 1/2 cup.

ORANGE

Nature: cooling
Actions: lubricates lungs, resolves mucus,

increases appetite, strengthens spleen, quenches thirst, promotes body fluids

Conditions: thirst, dehydration, stagnant chi, hernia

Folk Remedies:
1. <u>Cough with lots of mucus</u> – cook the orange and eat it.
2. <u>Stuck mucus, stagnant chi, chest fullness or distention</u> – make tea from dried orange peel.
3. <u>Chi stagnation, prostate enlargement and hernia</u> – make tea from orange seeds.

PAPAYA

Nature: neutral

Actions: strengthens stomach and spleen, aids digestion, clears summer heat, lubricates lungs, stops cough, aids irritability, kills worms, increases milk production

Conditions: cough, indigestion, stomachache, eczema, skin lesions, intestinal worms

Folk Remedies:
1. <u>Increasing milk production</u> – put fresh papaya in fish soup.
2. <u>Cough</u> – peel and steam papaya, then add honey.
3. <u>Stomachache and indigestion</u> – cook papaya and eat with or after meals.
4. <u>Intestinal worms</u> – sun dry green papaya, powder, and take 2 teaspoons on an empty stomach every morning.
5. <u>Skin lesions</u> – apply fresh papaya.

PEACH

Nature: very cooling

Actions: lubricates lungs, clears heat, aids diabetes, promotes body fluids, induces sweating

Conditions: diabetes, dry cough, intestinal worms, vaginitis

Contraindications: Not to be used with damp and cold conditions.

Folk Remedies:

1. Inducing sweating or killing worms – drink peach leaf tea.
2. Promoting blood circulation – make tea from the innermost seed, the kernel.
3. Dry cough – eat fresh peaches.
4. Vaginitis – douche with peach leaf tea.

PEAR (ESPECIALLY PEAR APPLE)

Nature: cold

Actions: regenerates body fluids, quenches thirst, calms the heart, lubricates lungs, relieves restlessness, promotes urination, clears heat, detoxifies, lubricates the throat, dissolves mucus, descends and cools cough

Conditions: cough (heat in the lungs), excess mucus, irritability, thirst, dry throat, hoarse throat, retina pain, constipation, difficult urination, skin lesions, alcohol intoxication

Contraindications: Not to be used with cold stomach and spleen, manifesting as cold extremities or diarrhea. Also, not to be used by pregnant women, or in cases of anemia.

Folk Remedies:

1. Cough and bronchitis – core the pear and steam it; eat 3-4 times daily. Pear can also be

cooked with scallions.
2. Acute voice loss - peel and juice 2-3 pears, adding 2 teaspoons of honey.
3. Whooping cough - core the pear and insert .5 grams of ephedra; steam, then remove the herb and eat the pear.
4. Nausea, belching - core the pear and insert 10-15 cloves; steam, then remove the cloves and eat the pear.
5. Alcohol intoxication - drink pear juice or tea to prevent hangover.

PERSIMMON

Nature: cooling
Actions: lubricates lungs, stops cough with heat, dissolves sputum, strengthens spleen, stops diarrhea, quenches thirst, clears heat
Conditions: pain in the throat due to heat, cough, thirst, vomiting blood, dysentery, alcohol intoxication
Contraindications: Do not eat persimmons along with crabs as the combination produces extreme diarrhea.
Folk Remedies:
1. Vomiting or coughing blood - cook a half ripened persimmon in rice wine for 10 minutes; eat the persimmon. Another remedy is to take dried, charred persimmon powder in warm water.
2. Bleeding ulcers and lower intestinal bleeding - take dried, charred, powdered persimmon in warm water (about a tablespoon of the powder).
3. Hypertension - drink 3 glasses daily of unripened persimmon juice.
4. Nausea and vomiting - add dried persimmon to water to make a mush, steam it and take 2

67

tablespoons 3 times daily for 3–4 days or until condition ceases. Cloves could be a good addition; or make persimmon cap and cloves tea.
5. Alcohol intoxication – take persimmon juice or tea.
6. Ulcerated skin lesions – apply a combination of charred persimmon powder and black pepper.

PINEAPPLE

Nature: hot and damp
Actions: clears heat, dispels summer heat, aids digestion, stops diarrhea
Conditions: heat stroke, irritability, thirst, indigestion, diarrhea
Contraindications: Pineapples are slightly toxic; this can be neutralized by washing with salt water.
Folk Remedies:
1. Heat stroke and irritability – drink fresh juice.
2. Nephritis (kidney inflammation) – make tea from peeled pineapple and reed roots; drink freely throughout the day.
3. Bronchitis – boil tea and add honey.
4. Dysentery – boil tea.

PLUM

Nature: slightly warming
Actions: stimulates appetite, aids digestion, regulates body fluids, stops thirst, softens or soothes the liver, removes stagnation of chi, removes the feeling of "steaming bones"

Conditions: dehydration, thirst, chi stagnation, erratic energy flow, poor digestion, dysentery
Contraindications: Too many plums are not good for the teeth.
Folk Remedies:
1. Dysentery – drink plum skin tea.

RASPBERRY

Nature: slightly warming
Actions: tonifies liver and kidneys, astringes essence, astringes urination
Conditions: kidney and liver deficiency, blurry vision, spermatorrhea, seminal emission, frequent urination
Folk Remedies:
1. Impotence and seminal emission – take dry raspberries, charcoal and grind to powder; take 3 teaspoons every night before bed with some rice wine.
2. Bed-wetting or frequent urination – take charcoaled raspberry powder, make tea and drink before bedtime every night.
3. Eczema, skin lesions, and fungus conditions – boil fresh raspberries to a concentrate; wash area with this.

STRAWBERRY

Nature: cooling
Actions: lubricates lungs, promotes body fluids, strengthens spleen, detoxifies in alcohol intoxication
Conditions: dry cough, sore throat, difficult

urination, food retention, lack of
appetite

Folk Remedies:

1. <u>Dry cough</u> – mash strawberries with brown sugar;
steam and eat 3 times daily.
2. <u>Dry throat, thirst, hoarse voice, sore throat</u> –
take 1 glass fresh strawberry juice 2 times
daily.
3. <u>Difficult urination</u> – mash fresh strawberries,
add cold water; drink 3 times daily.
4. <u>Lack of appetite, food retention, abdominal
distention and pain</u> – eat 5 strawberries before
each meal.

TOMATO

Nature: slightly cooling
Actions: promotes body fluids, quenches thirst,
strengthens stomach, aids digestion, cools
blood, clears heat, detoxifies, calms the
liver, removes stagnant food
Conditions: liver heat rising, hypertension,
bloodshot eyes, dehydration, indigestion due to low stomach acid, food
retention, kidney infection

Folk Remedies:

1. <u>Hypertension and eye hemorrhage</u> – take 2 raw
tomatoes on an empty stomach, every day for 1
month; also avoid spicy foods.
2. <u>Kidney disease</u> – eat at least 1 raw tomato per
day.
3. <u>Indigestion and food retention</u> – eat 1/2 – 1
fresh tomato after meals.

WATERMELON

Nature: cold
Actions: quenches thirst, relieves irritability, dispels summer heat problems, promotes diuresis, detoxifies
Conditions: sores, dry mouth, summer heat irritability, bloody dysentery, jaundice, edema, difficult urination
Contraindications: Not to be used in cold conditions or with weak stomach.
Folk Remedies:
1. Edema from nephritis - boil tea from the rind and the inner portion.
2. Jaundice - boil tea from the rind and red beans.
3. Fluid in the abdomen - make tea from the skins of watermelon, squash, and winter melon.
4. Constipation - boil tea from watermelon seeds or grind into meal and take with warm water.

GRAINS

BROWN RICE

Nature: neutral
Actions: strengthens spleen, nourishes stomach, quenches thirst, relieves irritability, astringes intestines, stops diarrhea
Conditions: indigestion, diarrhea, vomiting, nausea, "summer heat" irritability
Folk Remedies:
1. Bloody dysentery – cook brown rice with the persimmon "cap"; eat the rice.
2. Digestive aid – eat fermented rice cake after each meal.
3. Child regurgitating mother's milk – roast rice until overdone (brownish-black), add water and cook; give the child the fluid.
4. Diarrhea – grind rice, charcoal and take 1 - 2 teaspoons each time, 3 times daily.
5. Anorexia and digestive weakness – 1/2 c. over-done rice (bottom of pot) mixed with cardomon, fennel and orange peel.
6. Difficultly urinating – consume rice porridge continuously for one month.

BUCKWHEAT

Nature: neutral
Actions: descends chi, strengthens stomach, stops dysentery, lowers blood pressure
Conditions: chronic diarrhea, dysentery, spontaneous sweating, hypertension, skin lesions
Folk Remedies:
1. Skin lesions – boil tea and wash area. Or, roast

buckwheat, grind to powder and mix with rice
vinegar to make a paste; then apply to area.
2. Leukorrhea and chronic diarrhea – grind roasted
buckwheat, mix with warm water and take 2
teaspoons 2 times daily.
3. High blood pressure – make tea from buckwheat
and lotus roots.
4. Hemorrhoids – mix rooster bile with buckwheat
meal and roll in pill form. Take 1 t. twice
daily.

MILLET

Nature: cooling
Actions: stops vomiting, relieves diarrhea,
consolidates or astringes the stomach and
intestines, promotes urination, soothes
morning sickness
Folk Remedies:
1. Morning sickness and vomiting – eat millet
porridge as a regular staple; may add ginger.
2. Diarrhea – roast millet until aromatic; eat 1/2
cup 3 times daily.
3. Obstructed urination – boil tea from millet and
add 1/2 teaspoon brown sugar.
4. Diabetes – steam millet with yams and a few
dates.

OATS

Nature: warming
Actions: strengthens spleen, tonifies chi, harmonizes stomach, regulates chi, carminative,
stops lactation
Conditions: lack of appetite, indigestion,

abdominal distention and fullness, dysentery, swelling

Folk Remedies:
1. Stop lactation – boil sprouted oats tea and drink 1 cup 3 times daily, or use maltose as a sweetener in the diet.
2. Swelling – cook oats and azuki or mung beans to a mush.
3. Postpartum urinary and bowel obstruction – roast sprouted oats (malt), grind into meal, take 2 t. 3 times a day with lukewarm water.
4. Hepatitis – make tea from malt and dried orange peels, drink 1 c. 3 times daily.

PEARL BARLEY

Nature: cooling
Actions: promotes diuresis, strengthens spleen, benefits gall bladder, clears heat, detoxifies
Conditions: swelling, indigestion, diarrhea, jaundice, tumors
Folk Remedies:
1. For quitting coffee – substitute roasted barley tea for the coffee.
2. Swelling – cook soupy barley.
3. Heat conditions and skin lesions – blend barley and water, boil, and drink the liquid.
4. Skin lesions with pus discharge – sprinkle barley powder locally.
5. Acne – mix barley powder with aloe vera gel and make a facial mask to be applied every night before bed. Leave on overnight and wash off with water in the morning.

SWEET RICE

Nature: warming
Actions: warms spleen and stomach, tonifies chi, astringes urine
Conditions: stomach pains due to cold, diabetes, frequent urination, obesity, anemia
Contraindications: Eating too much will cause indigestion.
Folk Remedies:
1. Obesity – eat sweet rice cake (mochi); a small amount is very filling.
2. Indigestion – make tea from malt and sweet rice sprouts.
3. Anemia, lung tuberculosis – cook sweet rice porridge with red dates and pearl barley and eat regularly.
4. Spontaneous sweating – dry roast sweet rice and wheat bran, grind into meal; take 3 t. 3 times daily.
5. Stomach pains due to cold, diarrhea – make sweet rice porridge with yams, lotus seeds, Chinese red dates, and a pinch of pepper.

WHEAT

Nature: slightly cooling
Actions: clears heat, quenches thirst, relieves restlessness, promotes diuresis, calms spirit, stops sweating
Conditions: dry mouth and throat, swelling, difficult urination, insomnia, irritability, restlessness, menopause, spontaneous sweating, night sweats, diarrhea, burns
Contraindications: Always use organically grown wheat. Wheat absorbs 10 times

more nitrates (like from chemical fertilizers) than any other grain. This could explain the high incidence of allergies to modern day wheat.

Folk Remedies:

1. Insomnia, menopause, restlessness – make tea from 1 c. wheat, 12 grams licorice, and 15 Chinese black dates. Drink 1 c. 3 times daily.
2. Burns (initial stages) – make a paste of charcoaled wheat meal and sesame oil and apply locally.
3. Swelling, difficult urination – make tea from wheat and pearl barley.
4. Spontaneous sweating – make tea from wheat, crushed oyster shells and Chinese red dates.

SEEDS, NUTS & LEGUMES

ALMOND

Nature: neutral
Actions: ventilates lungs, relieves cough and asthma, lubricates intestines
Conditions: lung conditions, asthma, constipation, cough
Folk Remedies:
1. Cough and asthma - grind almonds to a fine meal, add fructose; dissolve 2 tablespoons in water.

AZUKI (RED) BEAN

Nature: neutral
Actions: strengthens spleen, benefits diabetes
Conditions: mumps, diabetes, leukorrhea, excessive thirst, hunger, or excretion of fluids
Folk Remedies:
1. Diabetes - after soaking red beans, boil 2 hours, drink the liquid 3 times daily.
2. Mumps - mash sprouted red beans and apply, either alone or mixed with dandelion.

BLACK BEAN

Nature: warming
Actions: tonifies kidneys, nourishes the yin, strengthens and nourishes blood, brightens eyes, promotes diuresis, and aids kidney deficiency
Conditions: lower back pain, knee pain,

infertility, seminal emissions, blurry
vision, ear problems, difficult urination

Folk Remedies:
1. <u>Beriberi</u> – cook black beans with carp.
2. <u>Spontaneous menopausal sweating</u> – make boiled black bean juice.
3. <u>Low back pain, weak knees, frequent urination, and other kidney weakness symptoms</u> – slowly cook (for about 2-3 hours) 1/2 cup black beans, 1/2 cup water, and 3/4 cup rice wine. This is a good winter tonic.
4. <u>Kidney stones</u> – add kombu seaweed to the above winter tonic.
5. <u>Bed-wetting</u> – include black beans in the diet regularly.

MUNG BEAN

Nature: very cooling
Actions: clears heat, detoxifies, quenches thirst, promotes urination, reduces swelling, aids edema in the lower limbs
Conditions: edema, conjunctivitis, diabetes, dysentery, "summer heat" problems, heatstroke, dehydration, food poisoning from spoiled food
Contraindications: Not for cold conditions.
Folk Remedies:
1. <u>Dysentery</u> – take 5 parts mung beans to 1 part black pepper; grind to a powder and take 1 tablespoon 3 times daily. Usually one will notice results in 6-12 hours. The black pepper acts as an anti-bacterial agent.
2. <u>Breast abscess and boils</u> – take 2 tablespoons mung bean powder 2 times daily.
3. <u>Hives and bad skin lesions</u> – make mung bean juice in the blender and drink raw.

80

4. Summer heat problems - make soup from mung beans, barley, and rice.

PEANUT

Nature: neutral
Actions: improves appetite, strengthens spleen, regulates blood, lubricates lungs, promotes diuresis, aids in lactation
Conditions: edema, lactostasis, blood in urine, insomnia, lack of appetite
Folk Remedies:
1. Edema - make peanut tea for 7 consecutive days.
2. Lack of milk - steam peanuts, mash, and add to soupy rice.
3. Chronic cough - combine peanuts, jujube dates, and honey; make tea and take twice daily.
4. Chronic nephritis - combine peanuts and red dates; make tea and eat the solids. Take for 1 week.
5. Insomnia - boil peanut tea, take in the evening.
6. Hypertension - take peanut shells and boil tea or grind into powder and take with warm water; take 3 times daily for at least 20 days.

PEA

Nature: neutral
Actions: strengthens digestion, strengthens spleen and stomach, promotes diuresis, lubricates intestines
Conditions: indigestion, edema, constipation
Folk Remedies:
1. Edema - roast peas until dry, powder and take with warm water.

2. <u>Indigestion</u> – make blender pea juice and take with meals.

PINE NUT

Nature: warming
Actions: lubricates lungs, stops cough, lubricates intestines, promotes body fluids
Conditions: dry cough, constipation
Contraindications: Not to be used in diarrhea, seminal emission, or any mucus conditions.
Folk Remedies:
1. <u>Dry cough</u> – grind walnuts and pine nuts, add honey and slowly cook over low flame until thick; take 2 teaspoons with warm water.
2. <u>Constipation</u> – eat pine nuts with rice porridge.

SESAME SEED

Nature: slightly warming
Actions: nourishes liver and kidneys, lubricates intestines, blackens gray hair, tonifies the body overall
Conditions: backache, weakness, premature graying, ringing in the ears, blurry vision, dizziness, constipation, dry cough, blood in the urine, tonic for older people, weak knees
Contraindications: Always grind sesame seeds because the tough cell wall makes them indigestible whole.
Folk Remedies:
1. <u>Weakness conditions</u> – use black sesame seeds, grind to a meal, mix with honey to make a paste;

take 2 teaspoons 2 times daily.
2. <u>Dry cough and asthma</u> – roast sesame seeds, grind
to a meal and add ginger juice and honey. Take 1
teaspoon 3 times daily.

SUNFLOWER SEED

Nature: neutral
Actions: subdues liver, lowers blood pressure,
relieves dysentery, resolves pus
Conditions: headache, dizziness, liver fire rising,
bloody dysentery, intestinal worms
Folk Remedies:
1. <u>Headache or dizziness</u> – grind the seeds and take
with honey and warm water before bed.
2. <u>Hypertension</u> – take sunflower seed meal with
celery juice.
3. <u>Bloody dysentery</u> – cook the seeds with water for
1 hour, add honey; drink the liquid and eat the
seeds.

SOYBEAN

Nature: cooling
Actions: clears heat, detoxifies, eases urination,
lubricates lungs and intestines, provides
an excellent protein food
Conditions: lung and stomach heat, dry skin,
ferocious appetite, stomach or mouth
ulcers, swollen gums, diarrhea,
constipation, general heat problems
Contraindications: Do not eat soybeans raw; they
can be toxic.
Folk Remedies:
1. <u>Heat conditions</u> – drink soy milk or eat tofu.

Soy milk is easily made by blending soaked soybeans with a larger volume of water; strain off the "milk" and bring to a boil for about 15 minutes; sweeten to taste. To make tofu curdle the soy milk with calcium sulfate, nigari, or lemon juice; strain and press the solids into a block.

2. Diarrhea – charcoal soybeans and grind to a powder; take 1 teaspoon 3 times daily.
3. Habitual constipation – boil tea from soybeans and drink 4 times daily.

WALNUT

Nature: slightly warming
Actions: tonifies kidneys, strengthens back, astringes lungs, relieves asthma, lubricates intestines, aids erratic, rebellious chi
Conditions: kidney deficiency, impotency, sexual dysfunctions, infertility, frequent urination, back and leg pain, stones in the urinary tract, cough, constipation, neurasthenia

Folk Remedies:
1. Impotency and kidney weakness – eat 20 walnuts a day for 1 month.
2. Back pain and cold type arthritis – take walnut meal with warm wine (preferably red wine).
3. Kidney stones – take 120 grams (approximately 2-3 cups) walnuts, grind to a meal and add 120 grams brown sugar; roast with sesame oil. Take 1/4 of the mixture 4 times a day.
4. Neurasthenia – take equal portions of walnuts, sesame seeds, and dried mulberries, mash together to a paste; roll small pills and take 3 pills 3 times daily.

MEAT, FISH, POULTRY & ANIMAL PRODUCTS

Please note, meat, fish and poultry are always used in cooked form and never eaten raw.

BEEF

Nature: warm
Actions: tonifies chi, strengthens spleen and stomach, dispels dampness, relieves edema, strengthens bones and tendons
Conditions: edema, abdominal distention and fullness, weak back and knees, deficient stomach and spleen
Contraindications: Not to be used with any type of skin lesions, hepatitis, or any type of kidney inflammation.
Folk Remedies:
1. Deficiencies of blood, chi, spleen — take cooked ground beef and soak it in water for 10 minutes; drink the juice.
2. Edema or chronic diarrhea — stew beef in water for 2 hours; drink the liquid.

CHICKEN

Nature: warming
Actions: tonifies chi, nourishes blood, aids kidney deficiency
Conditions: postpartum weakness, weakness in old people, cold-type arthritis, weakness after illness
Contraindications: Do not eat chickens that are force fed chemical pellets and injected with steroids and antibiotics. These type of chickens can cause a variety of

health problems, including sterility, early female puberty, disharmony in the menstrual cycle, male impotence, to name a few. Also, chicken is not to be consumed by those with heat type cancers such as leukemia, or when there are heat symptoms such as "burnt tongue".

Folk Remedies:
1. <u>Weakness or anemia</u> – cook chicken with tang kuei (Angelica sinensis). The darker meat birds such as the Chinese black chicken are the most tonifying.

CHICKEN EGG

Nature: cooling
Actions: nourishes yin, tonifies blood, stabilizes hyperactive fetus, lubricates dryness
Conditions: dry cough, hoarse voice, dysentery, blood and yin deficiency, hyperactive fetus
Contraindications: Eating too many eggs is not healthy. In general, do not eat eggs fried or raw.

Folk Remedies:
1. <u>Yin and blood deficiency</u> – steam the eggs.
2. <u>Postpartum</u> – eat eggs with green onions.
3. <u>Pain of dysentery</u> – cook eggs with rice vinegar.
4. <u>Hyperactive fetus</u> – eat a hard boiled egg daily.

FISH

Nature: warming

Actions: strengthens spleen, tonifies chi, removes dampness, regulates blood, aids diarrhea from spleen weakness

Conditions: low energy states, hemorrhoids, postpartum excessive bleeding, itching or exuding damp type skin lesions.

Contraindications: Do not eat fish raw, as it is often loaded with parasites. Always cook fish with garlic, ginger or onion to neutralize the potential toxins.

Folk Remedies:
1. Kidney deficiency and back pain – cook chicken with fish.

LAMB

Nature: hot

Actions: tonifies weakness, dispels cold, strengthens and nourishes chi and blood, promotes appetite, aids lactation

Conditions: kidney deficiency causing back pain, impotence, cold conditions, deficiency conditions, postpartum blood loss, lack of milk, leukorrhea

Contraindications: Lamb is generally not consumed in summer because of its hot nature. Not to be consumed in edema, malaria, common cold, toothache or any type of heat conditions.

Folk Remedies:
1. Anemia, weakness, blood deficiency– cook lamb with ginger and tang kuei (Angelica sinensis). In general, the meats are traditionally prepared with such herbs as tang kuei, jujube, astragalus, ginger, scallions, or ginseng for problems

of weakness and coldness.

MILK AND MILK PRODUCTS

Nature: neutral
Actions: strengthens weakness, nourishes chi and
blood, lubricates dryness
Conditions: nutritional deficiency, weakness,
malnutrition, anemia, constipation
Contraindications: Not to be used with damp or cold
conditions, or in cases of
diarrhea. In general not to be
used by adults or those who are
strong as dairy products can
then cause mucus and other
disorders. As an occasional
food used moderately, it should
not cause a problem; however,
not to be used daily.
Folk Remedies:
1. Weakness, malnutrition – give a glass of warm
milk.

PORK

Nature: slightly cold
Actions: moistens and nourishes organs, tonifies
chi, strengthens the middle burner
Conditions: internal dryness
Contraindications: Not to be taken by fat people,
those with deficient spleen and
stomach, hypertension, stroke
victims or those with diarrhea.

88

MISCELLANEOUS FOODS

ANISE

Nature: warming
Actions: strengthens stomach, regulates chi flow, harmonizes stomach, stops vomiting
Conditions: hernia, beriberi, abdominal pain, distention and gas, back pain and coldness, cold stomach
Contraindications: Not to be used in any type of heat conditions.
Folk Remedies:
1. Stomach pain due to coldness - make anise tea and add some wine.
2. Hernia - charcoal anise and grind to powder; add brown sugar and take with rice wine.

BASIL

Nature: warming
Actions: induces sweating, harmonizes stomach, antidote for seafood poisoning
Conditions: wind-cold, vomiting, diarrhea, seafood poisoning
Folk Remedies:
1. Common cold - boil tea from basil, ginger, and green onions.
2. Diarrhea, vomiting, seafood poisoning - boil basil tea.

BLACK FUNGUS

Nature: neutral, slightly toxic when raw

89

Actions: nourishes stomach, calms spirit, lubricates dryness, promotes blood flow,
removes stagnation
Conditions: blood stagnation such as tumor,
especially uterine, abnormal uterine
bleeding, bloody stools, hemorrhoids,
constipation
Contraindications: Not to be used by pregnant
women.
Folk Remedies:
1. <u>Hypertension, bloody stools, and hemorrhoids</u> –
take black fungus and dried persimmon, add some
honey, cook, and eat once a day.
2. <u>Abnormal bleeding, anemia</u> – boil tea from black
fungus and Chinese dates.
3. <u>Dysentery</u> – take 10 grams fresh black fungus
with warm water 2 times daily.
4. <u>Tumors of the visceras and female organs</u> – make
tea from black fungus and peach kernel, and
drink.

CAROB POD

Nature: warming
Actions: soothes and calms the spirit
Conditions: used as an alternative to chocolate,
and for caffeine addiction
Contraindications: Eating carob to excess will
cause agitation.
Folk Remedies:
1. <u>Chocolate substitute</u> – use powdered carob pods.

CINNAMON

Nature: hot

Actions: induces sweating, strengthens stomach,
warms any coldness in the body
Conditions: common cold, abdominal pain due to cold
stagnation, lack of appetite due to
cold stomach
Contraindications: Not to be used in any type of
heat condition.
Folk Remedies:
1. Postpartum abdominal pain - boil tea with
cinnamon and brown sugar.
2. Premenstrual syndrome, including lower abdominal
pain and bloating prior to menstruation - make
tea from cinnamon and hawthorn berries.
3. Gas pain in stomach area - grind cinnamon powder
and take with lukewarm water, 2 times daily.

FENNEL

Nature: warming
Actions: unblocks and regulates chi, strengthens
stomach, dispels cold, stops pain,
stimulates peristalsis
Conditions: stomachache, hernia, abdominal discomfort, coldness in the stomach
Folk Remedies:
1. Hernia - boil tea from fennel seeds, black
pepper, cinnamon, and orange peel. Externally
apply warming linament and heating pad.

GINGER

Nature: hot
Actions: promotes sweating, anti-toxin, antidote
for seafood poisoning
Conditions: common cold, cough due to coldness

(clear or white mucus), vomiting, diarrhea, cold type arthritis

Contraindications: Not to be used in heat conditions.

Folk Remedies:
1. <u>Colds, cough, vomiting</u> – make ginger tea.
2. <u>Diarrhea</u> – apply ginger plaster to the belly.
3. <u>Baldness</u> – rub fresh ginger on the scalp.
4. <u>Arthritis</u> – rub fresh ginger on painful areas and drink tea (not for heat type arthritis).

HONEY

Nature: neutral, unless heated, then it is warming
Actions: nourishes yin, lubricates dryness, tonifies weakness, harmonizes, antidote to drugs, strengthens spleen
Conditions: diabetes (small amounts), constipation, ulcers, dry cough, hoarse voice, burns, cold sores
Contraindications: Not to be used in diarrhea or conditions of dampness or phlegm.

Folk Remedies:
1. <u>Ulcers</u> – mix ginger juice and honey and take on an empty stomach every morning.
2. <u>Burns</u> – apply locally.
3. <u>Cough, constipation, and hoarseness</u> – mix honey with water and/or almonds.

Note: Try to avoid heating honey unless a warming nature is desired; heating lowers the nourishing and beneficial effects. The darker honeys are more tonifying and tend to sink to the lower parts of the body. The lighter honeys are better for upper body problems.

MOLASSES

Nature: warm
Actions: tonifies deficiency, strengthens spleen, lubricates lungs, stops cough
Conditions: stomach and abdominal pain, chi deficiency, cough
Folk Remedies:
1. Stomach or duodenal ulcers - take 2 teaspoons molasses in lukewarm water to stop pain.
2. Cough - dice carrots, mix with molasses and leave it overnight; take 2 teaspoons 3 times daily.
3. Bed-wetting - boil cinnamon and licorice tea, add 2 teaspoons molasses.

OLIVE

Nature: neutral
Actions: clears heat, detoxifies, promotes body fluids, quenches thirst, clears lungs, benefits the throat
Conditions: whooping cough, dysentery, sore throat, dehydration, laryngitis, thirst
Folk Remedies:
1. Cough and dry conditions- take olives raw.
2. Sore, dry throat and laryngitis- take 50 black, pitted olives and 3-4 cups of honey; heat over a low flame. Take 2-3 tablespoons 3 times daily, swallowing slowly.

RICE VINEGAR

Nature: warm
Actions: detoxifies, invigorates blood circulation,

inhibits bacteria, astringent, closes
pores

Conditions: preventative for common colds, prevents
invasion from external pathogens,
malaria, acute arthritis, vomiting,
nausea, intestinal worms, hypertension,
burns, fungus infestation, bones
caught in the throat, gum disease,
hives, hepatitis, lung tuberculosis,
lung abscess, bronchitis

Contraindications: Not to be used at the onset of a
cold as it will trap the
pathogens inside of the body.

Folk Remedies:

1. <u>Malaria</u> – mix 30–50 c.c. of rice vinegar with 2
teaspoons baking soda; take 2 hours before the
episodic attack of chills and fever.
2. <u>Acute arthritis</u> – boil 2 cups rice vinegar down
to 1 cup; add green onions and boil another 5
minutes. Soak gauze pad and apply to sore area
twice daily until condition improves.
3. <u>Nausea and vomiting</u> – mix equal parts of rice
vinegar and water and drink.
4. <u>Intestinal worms</u> – take rice vinegar with water
on an empty stomach.
5. <u>Hypertension</u> – soak peanuts in vinegar; eat 20
peanuts every morning.
6. <u>Burns</u> – apply undiluted.
7. <u>Fish bones in the throat</u> – slowly drink 1 cup
vinegar, then eat something hard like bread
crust.
8. <u>Gum disease</u> – rinse mouth often with undiluted
vinegar.
9. <u>Hives</u> – make ginger tea, add rice vinegar and
brown sugar; take twice daily.
10. <u>Hepatitis</u> – soak apple–pear in vinegar; eat
daily.
11. <u>Lung T.B.</u> – soak garlic in rice vinegar for 2–7
days; take 1 clove 2 times daily.

12. Lung abscess - boil garlic in vinegar; take 1-2 cloves daily.
13. Bronchitis - combine 10 mashed garlic cloves, 1 cup vinegar, and 2 teaspoons brown sugar; take 2 teaspoons 3 times daily.

TOFU

Nature: cooling
Actions: clears heat, lubricates dryness, promotes body fluids, detoxifies, strengthens spleen and stomach
Conditions: chronic dysentery, malaria, lung tuberculosis, anemia, leukorrhea, irregular menstruation
Folk Remedies:
1. Chronic dysentery - stir fry tofu with vinegar.
2. Malaria - stir fry tofu with vinegar; take 3 hours prior to the onset of symptoms.
3. Lung tuberculosis - combine tofu and the herb, alismatis; boil, and eat the tofu. Take daily for 2 months.
4. Anemia - take frozen tofu that has been thawed, mix with egg white, until the egg white has soaked into the tofu; cook and eat daily for 1 month.
5. Leukorrhea - steam tofu and brown sugar.
6. Irregular menstruation due to coldness - stew together tofu, lamb, and ginger.

WHITE FUNGUS (JELLY MUSHROOM OR WHITE TREE EAR)

Nature: neutral
Actions: clears lung heat, strengthens spleen and stomach, promotes body fluids, tonifies

chi, invigorates blood, lubricates intestines, relieves alcohol intoxication,
nourishes yin

Conditions: cough, dry lungs, bloody sputum, irregular menstruation, arteriosclerosis,
hypertension, alcohol intoxication,
blood stagnation, constipation

Folk Remedies:

1. <u>Lung problems, constipation, bloody sputum</u> –
soak white fungus 12 hours, add honey, and
steam. Drink the liquid on an empty stomach.
This is known as "silver ear soup".

2. <u>Arteriosclerosis, hypertension, eye hemorrhage</u> –
drink "silver ear soup" before bed.

3. <u>Weakness after long illness or loss of blood</u> –
slowly stew white fungus, 10 Chinese dates, and
either pork or chicken.

SECTION

Remedies For Common Conditions

ACNE

This condition is characterized by skin blemishes or pimples. It can occur at any point throughout the lifetime and is related to a hormonal imbalance. In Chinese terminology the skin is controlled by the lungs, and acne is commonly a condition of heat in the lungs. Thus, the Chinese approach to this condition is to cool the heat, cleanse the lungs, and also externally work on the healing process.

Recommendations: squash, cucumbers, watermelon, winter melon, celery, carrots, cabbage, beet tops, dandelions, aloe vera, mulberry leaves, carrot tops, lettuce, potato, cherries, papaya, pear, persimmon, raspberries, buckwheat, alfalfa sprouts, millet, brown rice, mung beans, plenty of water

Remedies:
1. Blend a cucumber, apply externally; leave on for 20 minutes then wash off.
2. Apply plain, low fat, no chemicals yogurt; leave on for 20 minutes then wash off.
3. Rub watermelon rind on the acne.
4. Apply aloe vera.
5. Eat watermelon or drink watermelon juice.
6. Drink dandelion and beet top tea.
7. Drink lukewarm water with 2 teaspoons of honey every morning on an empty stomach. This effectively lubricates the intestines. If one does not evacuate the intestines regularly, the toxins either end up in the liver or coming out on the skin.
8. Boil raspberries to a concentrate and wash area with it.
9. Roast buckwheat, grind to powder and mix with rice vinegar into a paste, then apply to area.
10. For oozing acne condition, cover area with

pearl barley powder over night, wash off with water; or, mix pearl barley powder with aloe vera gel into a paste and leave on area over night, then wash off with water.

11. Make tea from carrot tops, carrots, and beet tops, and drink.

12. For infected acne, apply dandelion poultice to the area.

Avoid: fried foods, fatty foods, spicy foods, oily foods, coffee, alcohol, sugar, smoking, stress, constipation, make-up, washing with chemicals or soap (wash with cool water), chocolate, ice cream, soft drinks, dairy foods, emotional stress, red meat, shellfish, bamboo shoots, white mushrooms

Note: If the face is dirty, steam it with hot water to induce sweating, then wash with cold water.

ALLERGY AND INTOLERANCE

Allergy is an acquired hypersensitivity to a substance that does not normally cause a body reaction. The allergenic substance may be pollen, smog, dust, certain chemicals in the air, chlorine, or certain food substances which elicit a sometimes violent body response. This condition is characterized by nasal congestion, tearing, sneezing, wheezing, coughing, itching, skin rash and eruptions, dizziness and nausea.

Recommendations: ginger, onions, garlic, bamboo shoots, cabbage, beets, beet top tea, carrots, leafy greens, yams, organic chicken gizzards

Remedies:
1. Drink ginger tea to induce sweating.
2. Drink beet top tea as a water source.

Avoid: wheat, citrus fruits, chocolate, shellfish, dairy products, eggs, potatoes, polluted meats, polluted air, and constipation

ANOREXIA AND BULIMIA

Anorexia is medically defined as a lack of appetite for food or a hysterical avoidance of food. This condition is particularly prevalent among young American women obsessed with being thin. There is usually an extreme loss of weight, no menstruation, fatigue, depression, and hypoglycemic patterns. Closely related to anorexia is bulimia, a condition in which one binges then purges, usually by vomiting. Emotional factors play a large part in both of these conditions.

Recommendations: bell pepper, cilantro, mustard greens, green onions, garlic, cinnamon, ginger, pumpkin, yam, beans, corn, barley, rice, persimmons, potatoes

Remedies:
1. For anorexia, prepare tea from green onions, garlic, cinnamon or ginger, to warm the stomach and stimulate digestive juices.
2. For anorexia, prepare soup from pumpkin, yam, beans, potatoes, corn, barley or vegetables.
3. For anorexia, prepare soupy rice.
4. For bulimia, give foods that bring rebellious chi down such as persimmons, cloves, potatoes, prune or plum tea, and mineral herbs such as oyster shell tea.
5. For anorexia, dry fry bell pepper and black pepper.

ARTHRITIS

Arthritis is an inflammation of the joints characterized by pain, redness, swelling, stiffness and hot sensation in the joints. Chinese medicine differentiates the following 4 types of arthritis.

1. Cold Type Arthritis

This type is characterized by sharp, stabbing pain in a fixed location and coldness in the joints. The pain is relieved by heat such as a warming linament, sunshine, or a heating pad. Usually this type individual would have a pale complexion.

Recommendations: garlic, green onions, pepper, black beans, sesame seeds, chicken, lamb, mustard greens, ginger, a small amount of rice wine (if individual does not have hypertension), 10-20 minutes of fresh air and sunshine daily, spicy foods, grapes, grape vine, parsnip

Remedies:
1. Rub garlic or ginger on the painful areas. Or moxa could be burned on ginger over the painful areas.
2. Drink scallion tea and rub on the painful areas.
3. Rub rice wine on the painful areas as well as consuming 1 shot glassful in the evening.
4. Drink grape vine tea added to red wine.
5. Make tea from parsnip, cinnamon, black pepper, and dried ginger.

Avoid: cold foods, raw foods, cold weather elements

103

2. Wind Type Arthritis

This type of arthritis is characterized by pain that shifts locations, comes and goes suddenly (much like the wind does), and sometimes causes dizziness.

Recommendations: snake meat (from non-poisonous ones), scallions, grapes (not wine), grape vine and mulberry vine tea, black beans, most grains, and plenty of leafy vegetables

Avoid: meats, shellfish, sugar, alcohol, smoking, and all stimulants

3. Damp Type Arthritis

This is characterized by heavy feeling extremities, stiffness, swelling, dull aching pain that lingers and sluggishness. Most obese people tend to be "damp".

Recommendations: barley, mung beans, mustard greens, red beans, millet, sweet rice wine with meals, cornsilk tea, diuretic foods and herbs

Remedies:
1. Cook together barley, mung beans and red beans.
2. Drink cornsilk tea freely.

Avoid: cold foods, raw foods, dairy products

4. Heat Type Arthritis

This is characterized by red, swollen, painful, hot joints, general disability, and usually acute onset.

Recommendations: plenty of fresh fruits and vegetables, dandelion, cabbage, mung beans, winter melon, soybean sprouts

Remedies:
1. Apply poultices of crushed dandelion greens, changing every 2 hours.

Avoid: spicy foods, alcohol, smoking, all types of stress, green onions

Note: Sometimes we observe 2 or 3 types of arthritis occurring simultaneously, such as cold, wind, and damp types together. In such cases, choose foods that aid each condition and are not contraindicated for any type present. Herbal therapy can be of great benefit in cleaning out the joints. Acupuncture is one of the most effective treatments for arthritis, although progress is sometimes slow.

ASTHMA

Asthma is characterized by wheezing or difficulty breathing due to the bronchials (branches) of the lungs becoming clogged with waste products, or constriction due to spasms, or swelling of the bronchials. Asthma may be triggered by an allergy to food, air pollution, cold air, heart weakness, previous lung damage, mental or physical fatigue, emotional disturbance, or hormonal imbalance. In the case of a weak heart, the heart is not strong enough to push the blood through the lungs to be oxygenated, and the blood back flows into the lungs. In this case there will be edema and bruising also.

Chinese medicine divides asthma into 2 types: hot type, characterized by rapid, coarse breathing, yellow, sticky mucus, fever, and red face; and cold type, characterized by white, clear, or foamy mucus, cold extremities, and pale face. The remedies listed would be useful to either type. During times of remission from asthma attack, one would seek to nourish the lungs and kidneys.

Recommendations: apricot kernels, almonds, walnuts, basil, carrots, pumpkins, winter melon, sunflower seeds, loofa squash, figs, daikon, litchi fruit, tangerines, loquats, honey, molasses, mustard greens, sesame seeds, placenta and umbilical cord*

*These particular substances are not so easily obtainable in America, and only those from a healthy mother source are desirable.

Remedies:
1. Egg yolk oil. This is made as follows: take 20 hard boiled egg yolks; slowly heat in a dry pan, mashing them until the oil comes out. When the

106

yolk has blackened, separate the egg yolk oil. Since it is very strong tasting, it is best taken in gelatin capsules, 2 after meals, 3 times daily. Continue this remedy for 15-30 days.

2. Mix 1/2 cup fig juice with 1/2 cup lukewarm water and drink daily.
3. Cut the top out of a small winter melon, remove the seeds, fill with molasses, close the top up with cheesecloth and steam. Consume daily for 7 days.
4. Take an unpeeled orange, stick a chopstick through it, roast until the peel blackens. Remove the peel and eat the insides; one orange daily for 7 days.
5. Bake squid bone until crisp; grind to a powder and take 1 teaspoon with honey daily for 7 days.
6. Drink apricot kernel tea.
7. Drink fresh fig juice 3 times daily.

Avoid: mucus producing foods, cold foods, fruits, salads, all shellfish, dairy products, watermelon, bananas, mung beans, salty foods, cold weather, and especially ice cream

CANCER

According to Chinese Medicine, cancer is an abnormal growth of tissue that results from some sort of stagnation, of chi, blood, mucus, or body fluids. The stagnation can be caused by some external irritant such as cigarette smoke or chemicalized foods or by strong emotions. When the body is irritated over a long period of time, it reacts to the irritant by growing to protect itself. However, at a certain point the cell growth becomes abnormal and uncontrollable and cancer cells result. Strong emotions lead to chi stagnation which in turn can lead to stagnations of blood, mucus or body fluids.

The Western approach to cancer is to kill the cancer cells with harsh chemicals, radiation, etc. However, these methods also intoxicate the healthy cells. The Chinese approach to cancer is to support the body so that it can combat the cancer cells itself. The cancer is considered to be a toxin in the body, thus a detoxifying diet is also utilized.

Recommendations: seaweed, mushrooms (especially Chinese black ones), figs, beets, beet tops, papayas, mung beans, licorice, sea cucumbers, carrots, garlic, walnuts, litchi fruits, mulberries, asparagus, pumpkins, burdock, dandelion greens, white fungus, taro roots, pearl barley, grains, plenty of fresh fruits and vegetables

Remedies:
1. Blend black or ling zhi mushrooms and white fungus, boil and drink the soup 3 times daily.
2. Boil together mung beans, pearl barley, azuki beans, and figs. This makes a delicious dessert that will aid appetite and sustain the energy

level.
3. Make tea from dandelion, burdock, and chrysanthemum flowers; you may also add beet tops or carrot tops. Drink this as the regular beverage every day.
4. Always wash commercially grown fruits and vegetables in salt water to neutralize the chemicals.
5. Take garlic and seaweed, slightly stir fried in water.
6. Drink carrot and celery juice.
7. Make blender juice from a mixture of fresh vegetables and take warm.
8. For breast cancer, make tea from asparagus and dandelion and apply poultice to breast.
9. For breast tumor, charcoal the pumpkin "cap" into powder; take 1 t. of powder in 1 shot of rice wine 2 times daily.
10. Make tea from seaweed (any variety), peach kernel and green orange peels. Externally for visible tumors, make poultice from seaweed, ginger and dandelion, and apply locally.

Avoid: meat (if patient cannot handle vegetarian diet a little fish could be eaten), chicken, coffee, cinnamon, anise, pepper, dairy products, spicy foods (except garlic), high fat foods, cooked oils, chemical additives, moldy foods, smoking, constipation, stress, and all irritations

CANDIDA YEAST INFECTION

This condition is becoming fairly common in modern society, primarily due to the widespread, long term use of antibiotics which severely weaken the immune system. Everyone has the candida yeast living in their bodies; however, only when disharmony and weakness occur do we have systemic yeast infections develop. The symptoms can include chronic fatigue, chronic infections, primarily in the skin, bowels, bladder, vagina, and throat; diarrhea or constipation, headaches, bloating, poor digestion, etc. When the immune system is weakened through overwork, too much sex, or stress, the candida flares up and the body can no longer control it.

Recommendations: dandelions, beet tops, carrot tops, barley, garlic, rice vinegar, mung beans, citrus fruits

Avoid: sugar, excessive fruits, yeast containing foods, processed foods, cheese, fermented foods, soy sauce, smoking, alcohol, caffeine, and constipation.

CATARACT

This is a condition that usually affects older people in which the lens of the eye becomes cloudy and there is decreased visual acuity. It may be accompanied by dizziness, vertigo, fatigue, lower back pain, etc. Western medicine treats cataract by surgically removing the lens.

Recommendations: chrysanthemum, cilantro, spinach, cloves, water chestnuts, yams, lycii fruit, black beans. Exercise the eyes regularly and get plenty of oxygen into the bloodstream.

Remedies:
1. Stuff nose with fresh cilantro and inhale the aroma; do this 3 times daily.
2. Cook spinach with no spices and eat daily.
3. Steam the eyes over boiling spinach.
4. Grind cloves into a very fine powder and add a little milk to make a ointment. Apply to eyes 3 to 5 times daily.
5. Make fresh water chestnut juice and use as an eye drop.
6. Make tea from clam shells, orange peels, lycii fruit, and chrysanthemum. Drink 3 times daily for at least 2 weeks.
7. Grind into powder: black beans, sesames, yams, and walnuts then add a little honey and eat 1 T. 2 times daily for 1 month.

Avoid: any type of spices (very important), salt, garlic, eye strain, constipation

CHRONIC BLADDER INFECTION

This is a common condition in women, characterized by painful or burning urination, the feeling that there is still urine left in the bladder after urinating; fever, low back ache. If this condition occurs in a man it is a warning sign of something more serious such as venereal disease or cancer. Women are prone to chronic bladder infections because of the short length of their urethra. In Chinese terminology it is a condition of damp heat.

Recommendations: watermelon, pears, carrots, celery, corn, mung beans, cornsilk, squash, wheat, water chestnuts, barley, red beans, millet, oranges, cantaloupe, grapes, strawberries, lotus roots, loquats, plenty of water, and in general cooling and diuretic foods

Remedies:
1. Drink watermelon and pear juice 3 times daily.
2. Drink carrot and celery juice 3 times daily.
3. Drink cornsilk tea freely.
4. Eat squash soup for at least 7 days.
5. Eat steamed lotus root and water chestnuts 2 times daily.
6. Drink blended mung bean juice.
7. Drink fresh strawberry juice.
8. Drink tea made from wheat and pearl barley.

Avoid: heavy proteins, meat, dairy products, onions, scallions, ginger, black pepper, alcohol

CHRONIC BRONCHITIS

This is a common condition in older people, commonly due to a lowered immunity. It often occurs during winter and spring. Main symptoms include cough, mucus, shortness of breath, and fullness in the chest.

Recommendations: carrots, apricot kernels, persimmons, white fungus, pears, honey, jellyfish, ginger, water chestnuts, yams, sweet potatoes, Chinese red or black dates, daikon radish, walnuts, papaya, peach kernels, lotus roots, seaweed, betel nut, white pepper, loquat leaves, lily bulbs, pine nuts, mulberry leaves, chrysanthemum, ginko, basil seeds, pumpkins, taro, winter melon seeds. Always try to keep warm.

Remedies:
1. Take carrots and apricot kernels cooked with rice porridge. Take 3 times daily for 30 days.
2. Take white fungus and rock sugar, steam and eat 2 - 3 times daily for 1 month.
3. Take 2 - 3 pears, remove core and fill with honey and eat before bed every day for 1 month.
4. Take jellyfish and water chestnut to make soup.
5. Take ginger, apricot kernel, pine nuts, and walnuts; mash, add rock sugar, and steam. Eat 2 - 3 T. twice daily for at least 14 days.
6. Make juice from pineapple and lemon; drink before meals for immediate relief.
7. Take 3 dried persimmons boiled in 2 c. water, reduced to 1 c., add some honey, drink 2 - 3 times daily.
8. Take daikon, add maltose and steam. Eat 2 - 3 times daily for relief within 1 week.
9. Take papaya, peeled, add honey and steam.
10. Grind seaweed into powder, add honey and make into pills and take 1 t. 2 - 3 times daily

after meals.

11. Boil tea from betel nuts, drink as your water for 1 month.

12. Take carrots, white pepper, ginger, and dried orange peels and make tea. Drink 2 c. daily.

13. Take 1 T. honey and 1 T. sesame oil, warm in pan and take for immediate relief.

14. Cut banana into small pieces and cook with rock sugar until sugar melts. Take 1 - 2 pieces of banana every evening for 1 week.

15. Use seed from such vegetables as daikon, basil, spinach, and make tea, adding honey.

16. Take 1 T. molasses and 1/2 T. raw ginger juice with warm water 2 - 3 times daily.

17. Use fresh, yellow chrysanthemum flowers and boil into a thick juice; take regularly.

18. Mash cooked taro root and add honey.

19. Take raw eggplant juice (especially good for blood in the mucus).

Avoid: overworking, getting chilled, stimulating foods, spicy foods, smoking, alcohol, caffeine, cold drinks

CHRONIC SINUSITIS

This condition is due to an acute inflammation of the nasal passages over a long period of time. There is often drainage or congestion, difficulty breathing through the nose, sometimes dryness of the nostrils, headaches, ringing in the ears, etc.

Recommendations: ginger, green onions, magnolia flower, bananas, garlic, black mushrooms, chrysanthemum flowers, orchids, mulberry leaves, apricot kernels. Get plenty of fresh air.

Remedies:
1. Make tea from magnolia flower, basil, ginger, and green onion; drink 3 times daily for at least 1 week.
2. Combine magnolia flowers and eggs, cook together and eat.
3. Make tea from mulberry leaves and chrysanthemums, then cook rice porridge in the tea and add apricot kernels.
4. Mash green onions, soak cotton balls and alternately put in nostrils after having washed them with salt water.
5. Make garlic juice, add olive oil and soak cotton balls and alternately put in nostrils after having washed them with salt water.
6. Cook black mushrooms into a concentrated soup, then slowly use a dropper to put drops into the nose.
7. Boil tea of mint, basil, and ginger. While boiling the tea, inhale the steam through the nose, 3 times daily for at least 2 months.

Avoid: extremes of exposure to weather elements, coffee, smoking, stress, picking the nose, polluted air and smog

COMMON COLD

There are two basic types or stages of colds. In Chinese terminology they are the "wind cold type" and the "wind heat type". They have different symptoms and different treatments.

1. "Wind Cold Type"
This type often occurs with a change in weather or when one is exposed to wind and cold. With a weak immune function these pathogens enter the skin. The symptoms could include chills, fever, no sweating, headache, body ache, stiff neck, and clear copious nasal discharge. This is often the first stage of a cold. When the pathogens are at this initial, superficial stage, we seek to sweat them out. A hot bath or dry sauna could be of benefit to start the sweating process.

Recommendations: ginger, garlic, mustard greens and seeds, grapefruit peel, cilantro, parsnip, scallions, cinnamon, basil, soupy rice porridge, and eating as little as possible so as not to burden the system with a lot of digestion.

Remedies:
1. Lightly boil for 5 minutes garlic, ginger, green onion, basil, mustard, or cinnamon, drink the tea; go to bed and prepare to sweat.
2. Drink cilantro and ginger tea.
3. Drink scallion and basil tea.
4. Make tea from dried grapefruit peel.
5. Make tea from mustard greens, cilantro and green onion.
6. Make tea from parsnip and ginger.

Avoid: shellfish, heavy proteins and fats, meats, all vinegars. Vinegar closes the pores and "traps the thief in the house".

2. "Wind Heat Type"

This type of common cold is characterized by high fever, some chills, sweating, sore throat, cough, headache, body ache, and yellow nasal discharge or sputum.

Recommendations: mint, cabbage, chrysanthemum flowers, burdock root, cilantro, dandelion, apples, pears, bitter melon, drink plenty of fluids, and get plenty of rest

Remedies:
1. Drink cabbage broth freely.
2. Drink cilantro and mint tea.
3. Drink mint, chrysanthemum and dandelion tea.
4. Drink mint, dandelion and licorice tea.
5. Drink burdock tea.

Avoid: shellfish, meats, vinegar, drafts, hot foods

CONSTIPATION

Constipation is a lack of regular evacuation of the bowels or difficulty in defecation. The resulting symptoms may include bloating, abdominal pain, abdominal hardness, and bad breath. We should evacuate at least once daily, with the optimal times energy-wise being from 5-7 A.M. Food takes about 6-8 hours to go from the mouth to the intestines. The longer the waste remains in the intestines, the drier it gets and the more difficult to pass. Strained evacuation leads to hemorrhoids. Regular enemas or colonics are not a healthy solution to the problem. It is best to set a certain time for evacuation and train the body to respond accordingly. Rubbing the belly in a clockwise direction 100 times can stimulate the peristalsis of the intestines. Breathing with the mouth open is also beneficial in stimulating a bowel movement.

Recommendations: bananas, apples, walnuts, figs, spinach, peaches, pears, pine nuts, sesame seeds, mulberries, grapefruit, yams, honey, azuki (red) beans, apricot kernel, milk, yogurt, alfalfa sprouts, beets, cabbage, bok choy, cauliflower, potato, Chinese cabbage, salt water

Remedies:
1. Eat 2 bananas on a empty stomach, followed by a glass of water.
2. Drink a glass of lukewarm water with 2 teaspoons of honey on an empty stomach.
3. Drink blended beets and cabbage on an empty stomach.
4. Make beet soup.
5. Eat 5-10 figs on an empty stomach, followed by a glass of water.
6. Drink a glass of lukewarm water with 2 teaspoons

of salt, on an empty stomach. This remedy should be used as a last resort when nothing else has worked and should not be used by those with edema or hypertension.
7. Eat a fresh apple on an empty stomach.
8. Drink mulberry juice.
9. Eat lightly steamed asparagus and cabbage at night before retiring.

Avoid: stress, tension, spicy foods, fried foods, meat, coffee

CORONARY HEART DISEASE

This is a condition in which the arteries that supply the heart become hardened and clogged, eventually leading to deprivation of oxygen and nourishment to the heart, thereby causing heart attack. Recent research has attributed the cause of coronary heart disease to faulty diet, obesity, continuous stress and tension, mental fatigue, hypertension, diabetes, low thyroid function, smoking, etc. Typical symptoms with coronary heart disease are dizziness, vertigo, palpitations, chest fullness, shortness of breath, pain in the chest area, irregular heart beat, spontaneous sweating, hardness in the lips and tongue, and angina when there is an obstruction.

Recommendations: American ginseng, brown rice, black fungus, sea cucumber, Chinese black dates, peanuts, vinegar, mushrooms (especially black), celery, seaweed, cassia seeds, lotus roots, jelly fish, chrysanthemums, hawthorn berries, water chestnuts, mung beans, pearl barley, peach kernels, ginger, soy sprouts, mung sprouts, other sprouts, wheat bran, buckwheat, persimmons, bananas, watermelon, sunflower seeds, lotus seeds, black sesames, wheat, garlic, green tea

Folk Remedies:
1. Take 3 grams American ginseng and cook with 1 c. brown rice and some rock sugar. Cook into a porridge and consume every morning.
2. Take black fungus and black mushrooms, soak over night then steam 1 hour and eat before bedtime.
3. Take sea cucumber, Chinese black dates and steam together. Eat every morning on an empty stomach.
4. Soak 10 - 15 peanuts in rice vinegar for 24 hours and consume in the morning both the

peanuts and the rice vinegar.

5. Cook tea from white or button mushrooms and Chinese black dates. Take 2 times daily for 1 month.

6. Make tea from seaweed, cassia seed, and lotus root; drink the tea and eat the seaweed and lotus root 2 times daily for at least 1 month.

7. Combine jellyfish, water chestnut, and rice vinegar; cook together into a soup.

8. Cook celery and yellow squash soup and eat once a day for at least 20 days.

9. Make tea from chrysanthemum flowers, hawthorn berries, and cassia seeds. Drink 1 c. 3 times daily for at least 20 days.

10. Take black fungus, pearl barley, and dried orange peel and boil into soup.

11. Grind betel nut and hawthorn berries; add rice flour, stir together and steam. Eat often.

12. Take 1 T. honey, 3 times a day.

13. Steam soy and alfalfa sprouts together and add some rice vinegar.

14. Slightly roast wheat and oat bran with black sesame and sunflower seeds. Sprinkle on vegetables or porridge.

15. Drink at least 2 c. green tea every day.

16. Go on a watermelon fast for 3 consecutive days.

17. Take peach kernel, safflowers, hawthorn berries, and make tea. Drink 2 c. daily for at least 1 month.

Avoid: fatty foods, stimulating foods, spicy foods, coffee, smoking, alcohol, simple carbohydrates (sugar, white flour, etc.), salt, stress, tension, worrying, emotional stimulation, lack of sleep

DIABETES

Diabetes is characterized by a high level of sugar in the blood and urine. Symptoms include excessive thirst, hunger, and urination. The Chinese refer to this condition as "exhaustion syndrome". Proper exercise is of utmost importance in stimulating normal glandular functions; exercises such as T'ai Chi Ch'uan, Chi Gong, or the 8 Treasures are particularly valuable.

Recommendations: pumpkin, wheat, mung beans, winter melon, celery, pears, spinach, yams, peas, sweet rice, soybeans, tofu, mulberries, squash, daikon radish, cabbage, organic pig or chicken pancreas, peach, millet

Remedies:
1. Eat a slice of pumpkin with each meal.
2. Make pumpkin and yam pie with no sweeteners.
3. Prepare soup from cabbage, yam, winter melon, and lentils.
4. Drink daikon, celery, carrot, and spinach juice.
5. Steam tofu, cool to room temperature, add sesame oil and slices of raw squash.
6. Make soup from mung beans, peas, and barley.
7. Drink chrysanthemum tea whenever thirsty.
8. Eat non-sweetened sweet rice cake or mochi between meals.
9. Steam millet with yam and a few dates.

Avoid: sweets, sugar, honey, molasses, smoking, alcohol, caffeine, spicy foods, and most raw fruits

DIARRHEA

This is characterized by the frequent passage of abnormally watery stools, usually caused by increased peristalsis, irritation of the intestines through improper diet, drugs, bacterial infections, parasites, or worms. This differs from dysentery in that diarrhea is generally due to digestive weakness, biological imbalance, and in general is a chronic condition. Dysentery, on the other hand, is caused by an infectious condition.

Recommendations: garlic, black pepper, blueberries, cinnamon, raspberry leaves, lotus seeds, burned rice, yams, sweet potatoes, fresh fig leaves, peas, buckwheat, litchi, guava peel, apples, charcoaled bread, ginger, pearl barley, basil, unripe prunes

Remedies:
1. Cook rice porridge with lotus seed and yams.
2. Eat burnt rice or bread.
3. Make tea from dried litchi and Chinese black date.
4. Take 2 T. dried apples, 3 times daily on an empty stomach with warm water.
5. Cook rice porridge with ginger and black pepper.
6. Drink black tea.
7. Take 2 bulbs of garlic, baked until black. Then boil in water and drink the tea.
8. Make tea from guava peel.
9. Make tea from ginger, fennel, basil, and Chinese black dates.
10. Cook rice porridge with pearl barley.
11. Make tea from unripe prunes.
12. Take sweet rice porridge.

Avoid: cold, raw foods, most fruits, juices, overeating

DYSENTERY

Dysentery is a condition of intestinal inflammation characterized by abdominal pain, intense, urgent, watery diarrhea with foul smelling, bloody or mucus feces, dry mouth, thirst, and decreased urination. To prevent dehydration, plenty of fluids should be consumed. The person will sometimes defecate 30 or 40 times daily. Food poisoning can be a possible cause. Dysentery is considered to be contagious, usually transmitted through unsanitary food or water. Sometimes the person also has vomiting.

Recommendations: buckwheat, sweet potatoes, peas, celery, scallions, taro root, ginger, garlic, carrots, daikon radish, green pepper, winter melon, cantaloupe, bitter melon, hawthorn berries, figs, Chinese prunes, pears, persimmons, guavas, olives, sunflower seeds, lotus roots, tea, soy products, corn, pumpkins, water chestnuts, squash, honey, mung beans, cherries, pineapples, watermelon, brown rice, oats, chicken eggs (only if chronic)

Remedies:
1. Take carrot juice mixed with a little ginger juice, honey, and green tea; drink 1 cup daily.
2. Make mung bean soup and drink throughout the day.
3. Take ginger, garlic, celery, and peas stir fried together; incorporate into regular diet.
4. Eat 4 persimmons daily.
5. Soak plums in rice wine for 3 days; take 10 plums 2 times daily.
6. Make sweet potato and pumpkin mush and have 3 times a day, for breakfast, lunch, and dinner.
7. Steam black tree fungus with a little sugar in about 1 1/2 cups of water.
8. Charcoal dried ginger, powder it, and take 1

teaspoon with soupy rice.
9. Drink prune tea before meals on an empty stomach.
10. Drink plum peel tea.
11. Cook brown rice with persimmon "cap" and consume the rice.
12. Consume eggs that are cooked with rice vinegar. This remedy is only appropriate for chronic cases of dysentery.

Avoid: dairy products, high-fiber foods, hard to digest foods, fried foods, meats, fish, raw foods, cold foods, chicken eggs (for acute cases of dysentery)

ECZEMA

This is a common skin condition that often affects extremities, genitalia, as well as other parts. The skin lesion is characterized by a raised spot that turns into a blister and eventually erupts, ulcerates and then forms a scab which is later sloughed off. It can cause extreme itching and pain.

Recommendations: potatoes, broccoli, dandelion, mung bean, seaweed, pearl barley, azuki beans, cornsilk, water chestnut, winter melon, watermelon

Remedies:
1. Mash fresh potato and apply locally, changing every 4 hours, for 3 days.
2. Apply honey to area.
3. Apply mashed daikon radish to area.
4. Internally, make tea from mung beans and pearl barley.
5. Make tea from dandelion and cornsilk.
6. Make tea from azuki beans, pearl barley, and cornsilk. Drink tea and eat the solids 3 times daily.
7. Boil soup from seaweed and winter melon, drinking at least once a day for 10 days.
8. Externally, wash with equal portions of salt and borax, dissolved in warm water; wash area 2 - 3 times daily.
9. Make tea from lily bulbs, Chinese black dates, and mulberries, drink 3 times daily for at least 10 days.

Avoid: external stimulation such as extreme weather condition of wind, cold, dampness, dryness, heat, etc., excessive sun exposure, chemical exposure, soap (use clean water to bath)

EDEMA/SWELLING

Edema is a condition of swelling due to abnormal accumulation of fluids in the cells. It can occur any place in the body, however, the common places that edema occurs are face, lower extremities, and abdomen. Abdominal edema can cause ascites and is usually related to liver dysfunction such as cirrhosis of the liver. The treatment chosen is to promote diuresis and ease urination. Heart, kidney, and liver are the organs that may be involved.

Recommendations: red (azuki) beans, corn, ginger skin, winter melon, winter melon skin, squash, apples, mulberries, peaches, tangerines, coconuts, seaweeds, fish (in general), celery, green onions, garlic, bamboo shoots, spinach, water chestnuts, millet, wheat, black beans, pearl barley, carrots, watermelon, oats, beef

Remedies:
1. Take fish, preferably carp, and cook into soup with azuki beans. Use 10 cups of water and cook down to 1 cup; consume only the liquid.
2. Take winter melon rind and azuki bean and enough water to cover; cook and eat 3 times daily.
3. Drink blended juice of apple, carrot, and green onion 2 times daily.
4. Boil tea from ginger skin.
5. Cook together pearl barley, mung beans, and azuki beans into a soup; consume 3 times daily. You may also add black beans to this soup.
6. Daily diet should be on the bland side, including plenty of vegetables and fish.
7. Eat plenty of watermelon, if it is summertime.
8. Drink coconut juice daily.
9. Cook oats and mung beans to a mush and consume until swelling subsides.
10. Cook and consume soupy pearl barley.

11. Drink beef stew broth.
12. Drink tea make from watermelon rind.

Avoid: rich foods, salty foods, lamb, stimulating foods, wine, garlic, pepper, shellfish, fatty foods, greasy foods

GLAUCOMA

This is an eye disease characterized by an increase in the pressure inside of the eyes. Its onset can be either acute or chronic. The sufferer often complains that lights have halos around them. The condition can progress to a point in which the pressure causes atrophy of the optic nerve, leading to blindness. During the onset there may be pain, headaches, nausea, vomiting, blurry vision, etc.

Recommendations: chrysanthemum, mint, oyster shells, mulberries, black sesame, betel nuts, lycii fruit, antelope horn, cassia seeds, grapefruit, lemons, oranges, carrots, beets, beet tops

Remedies:
1. Boil tea from mulberries, oyster shell, and black sesame, drink 3 times daily.
2. Make tea from chrysanthemum and mint, drink 2 times daily.
3. Boil tea from betel nut, drink 2 times daily.
4. Boil tea from cassia seeds, orange peels, beets, and lycii fruit, then use the tea to cook rice porridge; add a little honey.

Avoid: Self treatment is not usually recommended due to the seriousness of this condition. Seek professional guidance for close observation of the condition. Avoid visual stimulation, stimulating foods, alcohol, drugs, smoking, coffee, salt, drinking too much water.

HEADACHE

There are many different types of headaches, such as migraines, ones caused by muscular tension, hypertension, common cold, mental stress, hormonal changes, eye strain, etc. Each type of headache would have a corresponding treatment.

Recommendations: chrysanthemum flowers, mint, green onions, ginger, oyster shells, pearl barley, carrots, prunes, buckwheat, peach kernels

Remedies:
For headaches due to common cold or flu:
1. Make tea from ginger and green onions, boiling for 5 minutes; drink and try to sweat.
2. Steam aching portion of head over mint and cinnamon tea that is cooking, then dry head afterwards, avoiding catching a draft.
3. Make tea from chrysanthemum flowers, cassia seeds and drink.
4. Make buckwheat meal into a paste and apply to painful area until it sweats.
5. Drink green tea.
6. Make rice porridge and add garlic and green onions. Eat while hot, then get under covers and sweat.

For headaches due to high blood pressure, menstrual cycles, emotional stress or tension, or migraines:
1. Make carrot juice. If headache is on left side, squirt carrot juice into left nostril; if on right side, squirt into right nostril; if both sides are painful, squirt into both nostrils.
2. Take lemon juice and 1/2 T. baking soda mixed in a glass of water and drink.
3. Make tea of unripe green prunes, mint, and green tea.
4. Make tea of oyster shells and chrysanthemum

flowers, boiling for 2 hours.
5. Mash peach kernels and walnuts, mix with rice wine and lightly roast it; take 2 T. 3 times daily.
6. Rinse head with warm water, gradually increasing the temperature to hot.

Avoid: spicy food, lack of sleep, alcohol, smoking, excess stimulation, eye strain

Note: Menstrual type headache usually are accompanied by Premenstrual Syndrome (P.M.S.). Please refer to that section for further details.

HEMORRHOIDS

This is a common condition in America today, related to constipation. With dry stools the person strains to move the bowels and causes friction with the rectal tissues. Sometimes it can cause bleeding. Hemorrhoids can be due to overconsumption of alcohol, spicy or fried foods; lack of exercise; sitting or standing for too long; too much sex; pregnancy; or chronic constipation. A hemorrhoid is like a varicose vein in the rectum and can be very painful.

Recommendations: sea cucumber, black fungus, water chestnut, buckwheat, tangerines, figs, plums, fish, prunes, guavas, bamboo shoots, mung beans, winter melon, black sesame seeds, persimmons, bananas, squash, cucumbers, taro, tofu, cooling foods

Remedies:
1. Soak lower body in a warm bath to which has been added the tea of either mugwort, carrot tops, or figs. Bath should be warm enough to induce sweating and done daily.
2. Take black fungus with rice every morning for breakfast on an empty stomach; do this for 1 month.
3. Steam sea cucumber without salt or spices and eat for immediate pain relief.
4. Roast and grind black sesame seeds, take with warm water and honey every night before retiring.
5. Steam dried persimmons and eat.
6. Wash hemorrhoid with winter melon tea.
7. Boil papaya tea for 2 hours, without the skin, and soak area.
8. Grind mung bean powder, boil with dandelion greens and wash area with the tea.
9. Steam figs, add honey and steam again several

times, until it becomes soggy; consume every day.
10. Insert a raw potato suppository after each bowel movement.
11. Eat a banana everyday on an empty stomach.

For bleeding hemorrhoids, the following remedies can be used:
1. Take black ear fungus cooked with brown sugar; consume daily.
2. Every morning on an empty stomach, eat 3 bananas with some honey.
3. Before breakfast and after dinner every day for 2 weeks, eat a fresh squash.
4. Make taro root soup and eat regularly until bleeding stops and hemorrhoid heals.
5. Mash fresh plums and take with lukewarm water 3 times daily.
6. Wash area with hot water, then apply a cotton ball that has been soaked in garlic juice. Change cotton every hour.

Avoid: stimulating foods, spicy foods, alcohol, smoking, constipation, stress, lack of exercise, standing or sitting too long

HIVES

Hives is a skin condition which is characterized by an intermittent attack of extreme itching which results in welts, mostly on the arms, legs, back, and face. These elevated spots can spread throughout the entire body with scratching. It may be brought on by an exposure to wind or after consumption of shellfish. This condition in Chinese Medicine is considered invasion of wind.

Recommendations: winter melon rind, chrysanthemum, vinegar, papaya, ginger, Chinese black dates, dried prunes, black sesame, black beans, litchi, pearl barley, cornsilk, soybeans, mung beans, licorice, hawthorn berries, peach kernels, maple leaves, Chinese black mushrooms, mint leaves

Remedies:
1. Externally, take a sea salt bath, and rub salt on the hives.
2. Boil a thick tea from fresh maple leaves for an external wash of hives.
3. Internally, drink tea made from 15 g. gypsum, 9 g. hawthorn berries, 60 g. black beans, some winter melon rind and chrysanthemum flowers. Add some honey and drink 3 times daily.
4. Cook together papaya, ginger, and rice vinegar until vinegar is dried up. Eat the ginger and papaya 2 times daily for at least 10 days.
5. Mix honey with rice wine and steam. Drink 2 T. on an empty stomach every morning.
6. Cook together black sesame, black bean, and Chinese black dates and eat at least once daily.
7. Make tea of dried litchi, add some brown sugar and take 3 times daily.
8. Make tea of lotus seeds and 1/2 t. pearl powder.
9. Make tea of cornsilk and pearl barley and drink

2 times daily for at least 10 days.
10. Take equal portions of mung and soy beans, grind into powder, add water, strain and drink 1 c. 2 times daily.
11. Make tea of licorice, mung beans, and gypsum; drink 3 times daily for at least 3 days.
12. Eat 2 - 3 dried prunes daily.

Avoid: shellfish, allergic foods

HYPERTENSION

Hypertension, or high blood pressure, is characterized by wiry and rapid pulse, headache, dizziness,
tinnitus, blurry vision, palpitations, chest
tightness or fullness, fatigue, insomnia, vertigo,
and numbness of the extremities. It is commonly
caused by hardening of the arteries, kidney
dysfunction, or liver dysfunction. The normal
range of blood pressure is between 70 - 85 mm Hg
for diastolic and 100 - 135 mm Hg for systolic
measurement.

Recommendations: celery, spinach, garlic, bananas,
sunflower seeds, honey, tofu, mung beans, bamboo
shoots, seaweed, vinegar, tomatoes, water chestnuts, corn, apples, persimmons, peas, buckwheat,
jellyfish, watermelon, hawthorn berries, eggplant,
plums, mushrooms, lemons, buckwheat

Remedies:
1. Drink warm celery juice 3 times daily.
2. Eat 2 raw tomatoes on an empty stomach every day
   for a month.
3. Drink water, vinegar and honey regularly.
4. Drink chrysanthemum and spinach tea regularly.
5. Drink cornsilk tea.
6. Sleep on a pillow of chrysanthemum flowers to
   draw the heat out of the head.
7. Make mung bean soup.
8. Take garlic oil capsules to clean out the
   arteries. The capsules have the advantage of
   not overly stimulating the taste buds in the
   warming direction. The taste buds start the
   functions of many physiological processes; the
   spicy flavor can be too stimulating, in general,
   for hypertensive individuals.
9. Steam or bake jellyfish about 12 minutes, add
   vinegar, soy sauce, and sesame oil; take daily

for about 2 months.
10. Steam tofu, cool to room temperature, add vinegar and sesame oil. This can be combined with soupy rice for a nutritious breakfast.
11. Make lotus root tea and drink 3 c. daily for one month.
12. Make tea from chrysanthemum flowers and cassia seeds and drink daily.
13. Steam white fungus for 2 hours and take before bed time.
14. Drink hawthorn berry tea continuously for a long period of time.
15. Make soup from abalone and seaweed.
16. During the summer months, make watermelon juice or eat watermelon every day.
17. Make tea from watermelon rind, mugwort, and mulberry branches, drink 3 c. daily for 2 months.
18. Take celery, white onion (sweet), garlic, water chestnuts, and tomatoes and 4 c. water; boil down to 1 c. and drink every night before bed.
19. Take seaweed, pearl barley and a little honey and cook into soup; eat every day for 5 days.
20. Mix pig bile and mung bean powder; take 1 t. twice daily for at least 8 days.
21. Take black or white mushrooms and cook soup daily.
22. Eat 3 apples daily.
23. Drink organic banana peel tea.
24. Make tea from one peeled lemon, 10 fresh water chestnuts, and 2 1/2 c. water.
25. Drink 3 glasses daily of unripened persimmon juice for 1 week.

Avoid: smoking, alcohol, spicy foods, coffee, caffeine, all stimulants, fatty foods, fried foods, salty foods, stress, constipation, potatoes, strong emotions, pork, overeating, and low levels of calcium in the body.

Note: For low calcium levels make tea from shells (oyster, abalone, etc.) or fossils (dragon bones and teeth); strain and drink.

HYPOGLYCEMIA

This is a very common condition in America due to the stressful lifestyle and heavy sugar laden diet. Hypoglycemia is characterized by low blood sugar (the crash after the high), chronic fatigue, nervousness, shakiness, headaches, fatigue when hungry, irritability or faintness if meal is late, sweet craving, waking at night hungry, night sweats, light-headedness, mood swings, depression, and difficulty concentrating.

Recommendations: sweet rice, brown rice, yams, potatoes, walnuts, tofu, soybeans, corn, fish, chicken, vegetables, black beans, nuts (a good snack between meals), mild exercise, regular meal schedule, 4-5 small meals daily

Avoid: simple carbohydrates such as white flour and sugar, honey, fructose, maple syrup, fruits (eat very sparingly), coffee, smoking, fatty foods, fried foods, all stimulants

IMPOTENCE

This is a weak condition, most likely due to a nervous weakness, excessive stress, worrying, tension, physical fatigue, frequent masturbation, or excessive indulgence in sex. Impotence is characterized by not being able to have an erection when there is a desire to have intercourse, and there may be premature ejaculation. Other symptoms may include dizziness, insomnia, excessive dreams, low appetite, back pain, lower extremities weakness, knee pain, fatigue, etc.

Recommendations: scallions, scallion seeds, lamb, sea cucumber, shrimps, rooster, bitter melon seeds, ginseng, black beans, kidney beans, yams, lycii fruit, maintaining a calm composure

Tonifying foods are needed, thus, many of the remedies include meat, however, it does not have to be treated with meat.

Remedies:
1. Make lamb stew with daikon radish and Chinese black dates. Drink the broth and eat the lamb.
2. Make cake from black (red) sweet rice, black sesame, black fungus, lotus seeds, walnuts, and black beans. Eat with 1/2 glass of red wine.
3. Steam a rooster with ginger.
4. Take dried shrimps, sea cucumber, and fennel, and dry roast and grind into a powder and take 1 t. 3 times daily with rice wine.
5. Roast and grind bitter melon seeds, take 1 t. 3 times daily with rice wine.
6. Make tea from walnuts, lotus seeds, pearl barley, Chinese black dates, and lycii fruit, and drink 3 times daily.
7. Take 50 grams of chopped ginseng and 1/2 bottle of white liquor (like vodka or gin), seal

bottle, shake bottle daily and preserve for 1 month. Drink 1 shot every night with dinner for at least 20 days.
8. Cook together scallions, shrimp, and egg and take with a shot of white liquor.

Avoid: obscene visual stimulation, dairy products, sweets, masturbation, overwork, too much sex

INDIGESTION

This is a condition of poor digestion due to weak stomach, lack of digestive enzymes, or eating too fast. This causes a stagnation of food in the stomach, resulting in abdominal fullness or distention, bloating, and sometimes diarrhea due to insufficient digestion.

Recommendations: hawthorn berries, papayas, sweet potatoes or yams, figs, pineapples, brown rice, oats, pearl barley, sweet rice, daikon radish, black sesame seeds, apples, oranges. It is important to eat slowly and chew the food properly; digestion begins in the mouth.

Remedies:
1. Age orange peel for about 1 month. Boil tea and take after meals or simply suck on the peel for indigestion.
2. Eat papaya 2 times daily, in any form, raw, cooked, or dried.
3. Eat sweet potato cooked with brown sugar and water. In the last 3 minutes of cooking this mush, add some rice wine. Eat regularly for 2 weeks to improve digestion.
4. Blend daikon radish juice and take after meals.
5. Roast black sesame seeds with salt and take with warm water.
6. Eat a leaf of fresh mugwort, or blend into a juice.
7. Take apple, lemon, or orange juice after meals.
8. Eat an apple after each meal.
9. Consume 1/2 c. of overdone rice (from bottom of pan) mixed with cardamon, fennel and orange peels.
10. Make tea from sweet rice sprouts and malt.

Avoid: rich foods, fatty foods, greasy foods,

tension and stress while eating, reading the
newspaper or watching television while eating as
this takes energy away from digestion.

KIDNEY WEAKNESS

This is a common ailment among Americans, characterized by weakness and lack of energy. In Chinese medicine the kidney system involves much more than just filtering water. It also includes storing the essence of life (sperms and eggs); controlling bone marrow and the brain (called the "sea of marrow"); growth, maintenance, and reproduction; controlling bones; producing blood; and opening to the ear. The adrenal function is included in the kidney system; thus adrenal exhaustion is kidney exhaustion. Weakness of the kidneys often manifests in the back, knees, ears, or reproductive functions. Good kidney function is clearly of great importance to good health. Kidney function (and resulting problems) can be divided into kidney yang and kidney yin.

1. Kidney Yang Deficiency

This is characterized by impotence, infertility, coldness, swollen extremities, swollen face, frequent urination, premature ejaculation, diarrhea, low sexual drive, low energy, fatigue, pale face and tongue, low back pain, knee pain or weakness, deafness, ringing in the ears, and a general feeling as though the "fire of life is about out".

Recommendations: warming foods, chicken, lamb, scallions, sesame seeds, fish, baked tofu, soybeans, walnuts, eggs, lentils, black beans, lotus seeds, a little wine, ginger, cinnamon bark tea

Avoid: cold foods, fruits, raw foods

144

2. Kidney Yin Deficiency

In this condition there is not enough water to cool the fire so it manifests as heat symptoms. These may include irritability, insomnia, red cheeks, night sweats, low afternoon fever, damp palms, damp soles of the feet, dry mouth, low back pain, seminal emissions, ear ringing, red tongue, and blurry vision. 95% of the time kidney yin deficiency occurs in thin people since yin corresponds to substance.

Recommendations: cooling foods, mulberries, apples, peaches, pears, fresh vegetables, most beans, soybeans, tofu, soy sprouts, chrysanthemum flowers

Avoid: hot foods, spicy foods, smoking, alcohol, stress, and strong emotions

MASTITIS

This is an inflammation of the mammary glands, often occurring 3 - 4 weeks after delivery. It is a very common condition, resulting from an obstructed mammary duct and accompanied by a bacterial infection. There may be distention of breast, pain, swelling, redness on the surface, fever, etc. As the condition progresses, the symptoms may worsen and the patient may have chills, fever, increase in white blood cell count, swollen and painful lymph glands in the armpits, pus, ulceration of breast, etc.

Recommendations: cooling foods such as cabbage, cucumber, dandelion, lettuce, malt, reed root, lotus root, honeysuckle. It is important to keep the affected breast clean.

Remedies:
1. Make tea from malt (sprouted oat), drink 3 times daily.
2. Externally, take egg white mixed with green onions and apply to the area, changing 2 - 3 times daily.
3. Make tea from dandelion and honey, drink 3 times daily for at least 5 days.
4. Make tea from honeysuckle, mint, and licorice, drink tea and apply the solids locally.
5. Boil dandelions into tea then condense into a syrup and add to rice porridge. Eat 3 times daily for 5 days.
6. Combine cabbage, lettuce, and dandelions to make a poultice for external application.

Avoid: spicy, stimulating foods, coffee, smoking, alcohol, dairy products (especially if there is pus), breast feeding

MENOPAUSE

This is the time when a woman stops menstruating completely, usually occurring between 45 and 50 years of age. It may occur slowly or suddenly. Symptoms may include hot flashes, weakness, depression, emotional instability, lack of concentration, irritability, headaches, insomnia, night sweats, etc.

Recommendations: black beans, sesame seeds, soybeans, walnuts, lycii fruit, mulberries, yams, licorice, Chinese black dates, lotus seeds, chrysanthemum flowers. Try to remain calm.

Remedies:
1. Cook black beans with rice into porridge, eat 2 times daily.
2. Roast sesame seeds and add to rice porridge for breakfast.
3. Steam chicken with lycii fruit and yam.
4. Make tea from chrysanthemum and cassia seeds and take 3 times daily.
5. Take walnuts, lotus seeds, and sunflower seeds and make a porridge with rice.
6. Stew millet, mulberries, lamb, and lycii fruit.
7. Make tea from licorice, Chinese black dates, and wheat chaff (the part that floats on the surface when put into water). This will help extreme mood swings and depression.

Avoid: stress, tension, stimulants

MORNING SICKNESS

This is characterized by nausea and vomiting and affects some women during the first few months of pregnancy, usually clearing up after the third month. It occurs particularly in the morning, although in serious cases, it may last all day. Accompanying symptoms may include headache, dizziness, and exhaustion. One should seek treatment right away as it will affect nourishment to the fetus.

Recommendations: lentils, grapefruit peel, carp, ginger, orange peels, bamboo shavings, persimmon "cap", millet

Remedies:
1. Grind lentils into powder then take 2 T. with rice porridge, 3 times daily.
2. Make tea from ginger and grapefruit peel, drink 3 times daily.
3. Steam carp with ginger and cardomon for 30 minutes. Eat daily for at least 1 week.
4. Make tea from ginger, orange peels, and a little bit of brown sugar.
5. Take the "cap" off the persimmon, make tea and drink 3 times daily.
6. Make fresh scallion juice and fresh ginger juice and add a little bit of sweetener. Take 2 - 3 t. 3 times daily.

As soon as the morning sickness stops, discontinue the remedies.

Avoid: overeating, heavy meats

MOUTH SORES (ULCERS)

This condition is sometimes called herpes simplex. It is basically an ulceration on the mouth. One may experience pain, hot sensation, irritability, insomnia, headache, dizziness, palpitations, bad breath, etc.

Recommendations: mung beans, daikon, carrots, lotus root, persimmon "caps"

Remedies:
1. Make juice from carrots and lotus root and rinse the mouth 3 - 4 times a day for at least 4 days.
2. Take 5 - 6 persimmon "caps" and boil tea. When cool, rinse mouth 4 - 5 times a day.
3. Apply honey to local area to help heal faster.
4. Char eggplant into ashes, powder and mix with honey. Apply to the sores.
5. Boil mung beans soup and eat on an empty stomach.
6. Grind mung beans into powder, mix with honey; apply to area.
7. Rub sea salt on the sores, 3 times a day for 2 days. Also rinse mouth with salt water.

Avoid: spicy foods, stimulating foods, smoking, stress, alcohol, coffee, constipation

NEPHRITIS (ACUTE)

This is an acute kidney infection. This condition is characterized by some type of infection that precedes the condition, such as laryngitis, tonsillitis, scarlet fever, perisyphilus, mumps, etc. There may be swelling beginning in the face area then spreading throughout the body in about 2 days, followed by blood in the urine, hypertension, headache, dizziness, fatigue, malaise, low appetite, nausea, vomiting, and scanty urination.

Recommendations: black beans, mung beans, azuki beans, pearl barley, garlic, carp, winter melon, watermelon, watermelon rind, reed root, cornsilk, sweet rice, lotus root, water chestnuts

Remedies:
1. Cook soup with azuki beans, winter melon rind, water melon rind and cornsilk. Drink at least 3 - 4 times daily.
2. Make tea from lotus root, drink 4 large glasses daily.
3. Do a watermelon fast or eat lots of watermelon.
4. Cook soup with carp, azuki beans, winter melon, and green onions. Start with 5 c. water and cook down to 3 c. Drink the soup and sweat.
5. Make tea from cornsilk, cooking for 1 hour, then strain and cook again until almost dry, then add some fructose powder. Then take 1 T. 3 times daily dissolved in warm water.
6. Cook rice porridge with pearl barley, black bean and water chestnuts.
7. Make juice from carrots, celery, cucumbers, and squash.

Avoid: stimulating (sour, spicy, salty) foods, alcohol, caffeine, smoking, overworking, high protein foods

NEPHRITIS (CHRONIC)

This can result from acute nephritis that is not properly taken care of; or, a low immunity, causing kidney infection. The symptoms include swelling, hypertension, hyperprotein urea, fatigue, headache, dizziness, and achiness. If this condition does not get taken care of, over a period of time it can cause damage to the kidney, leading to uremia.

Recommendations: ginger, Chinese black dates, sweet rice, soybeans, winter melon, carp, yams, mung beans, black beans

Remedies:
1. Make rice porridge and add ginger, cinnamon, and Chinese black dates; eat for breakfast and dinner.
2. Remove the internal organs of a duck and stuff it with 4 - 5 cloves of garlic, then cook in soup. Do not add salt. Drink the broth and eat the duck every other day.
3. Cook carp with soy beans, winter melon, and green onions into soup. Eat once a day for at least 20 days.
4. Cook rice porridge with yams and eat for breakfast and dinner.
5. Steam together crab, garlic, and white wine, and eat once daily for 15 days.
6. Boil tea from cornsilk, winter melon rind, water melon rind, and azuki beans.
7. Crush entire watermelon (with rind) and slowly cook to a thick syrup. Take 2 T. syrup in warm water 3 times daily.

Avoid: stimulating (sour, spicy, salty) foods, alcohol, caffeine, smoking, overworking, high protein foods

PREMENSTRUAL SYNDROME (P.M.S.)

P.M.S. is a condition that occurs during ovulation or before menstruation, due to hormonal fluctuations. It may be characterized by abdominal cramps, bloating, backache, headache, tension, irritability, low energy, and mood swings. A healthy woman should have little or no discomfort during this time, however, approximately 70% of American women suffer from these symptoms. This is partially due to the large consumption of cold foods and drinks in this country that in turn cause the blood to stagnate. In Chinese terminology, P.M.S. is a condition of disharmony in the blood: either stagnant blood, not enough blood, or heat in the blood. Acupuncture, acupressure, herbs, diet, and Chi (Qi) Gong exercises are all very beneficial for relieving the symptoms and correcting the disharmony.

Recommendations: At least one week prior to ovulation or the usual onset of P.M.S. symptoms, regularly consume the following: ginger, green onions, fennel, orange peel, spinach, walnuts, hawthorn berries, cinnamon, and black pepper.

Remedies:
1. Make tea from ginger, green onions, fennel, black pepper, and orange peel, boiling for 10 minutes. Drink 3 times daily, starting at least 1 week before usual onset of P.M.S. symptoms.
2. Make spinach soup, boiling for 30 minutes.
3. Make hawthorn berry and cinnamon tea.

Avoid: cold foods, raw foods, excessive consumption of fruit, vinegar, all shellfish, coffee, stimulants, sugar, dairy products, and smoking

PROSTATE PROBLEM

This condition generally effects older men (over 40). As the man ages the prostate can become swollen and the urethra and bladder become less elastic. Thus, symptoms usually include difficulty urinating or dribbling.

Recommendations: pumpkin seeds, anise, tangerines, cherries, figs, litchis, sunflower seeds, mangos, seaweeds

Remedies:
1. Roast pumpkin seeds or boil into tea and incorporate into the daily diet.
2. Make tea from rhubarb, peach kernels, winter melon seeds, pearl barley, azuki beans, and cornsilk; drink 3 times daily.
3. Boil fig tea.

Avoid: dairy products, rich foods, fatty foods, greasy foods, all stimulants such as alcohol, caffeine, and smoking, stress, tension, and particularly avoid sex

PSORIASIS

This is a common skin condition, usually geneti-
cally inherited, characterized by pink or dull red
lesions with silvery scalings. The skin may
become very rough and scaly and may temporarily
improve, although it is usually a chronic type of
condition. When the scaling takes place one can
also see reddish dots under the skin, accompanied
by various degrees of itching and discomfort. It
can affect any part of the body, and is usually
worse during the winter time. In Western medicine,
there is presently no treatment for psoriasis.

Recommendations: unripened dry prunes, guava
skins, pearl barley, vinegar, garlic, walnuts,
cucumber, beet tops, dandelions, squash, mung beans

Remedies:
1. Take 15 peeled and sliced water chestnuts and 1
   c. vinegar (preferably aged rice vinegar),
   slowly simmer in a non-metal pot for 20 minutes
   until water chestnuts absorb most of the
   vinegar. Then mash into a paste and seal in a
   jar. Spread evenly on a gauze pad and apply to
   affected area, changing daily if not too
   serious, 3 times daily if serious condition.
   Mild cases should show improvement within 5
   days; serious conditions may take 2 weeks.
2. Take dried unripe prunes, remove pits, and
   simmer into a tea, then condense into a syrup.
   Take 2 T. in warm water, 3 times daily.
3. Take peel from guava, char and powder it, mix
   with sesame oil into a paste and apply 2 times
   daily for 1 week.
4. Apply mashed garlic to the affected area,
   changing 2 times daily for 1 week.
5. Make porridge from lily bulb, gypsum, and rice.
   Eat once daily for at least 10 days.

6. Take mashed walnuts, use cotton to absorb the oil, apply the pulp 3 times daily.

Avoid: spicy food, stimulating food, alcohol, caffeine, smoking, excessive sun exposure

SEMINAL EMISSION (SPERMATORRHEA)

There are 2 types of this condition. The first type happens when one has a dream and then ejaculates during sleep, also known as a wet dream. The other type is when one has ejaculation without a dream, either during sleep or during waking hours. One may also have dizziness, back pain, leg pain, weakness, palpitations, shortness of breath, lethargy, fatigue, etc. These symptoms point to a weakness which if not dealt with can lead to degeneration.

Recommendations: lotus seeds, sea cucumber, yams, dried ginger, scallions, pearl barley, black beans, shrimps, seaweeds, cold showers daily

Remedies:
1. Steam scallions with shrimp and rice wine. Eat daily for at least 15 days or until condition improves.
2. Cook soup from sea cucumber, seaweed, and black beans. One can add walnuts also.
3. Cook sea cucumber with rice porridge and eat for breakfast every morning.
4. Cook pearl barley, black beans, walnuts, and scallions to make a porridge; eat every morning for breakfast.
5. Make tea from ginseng, Chinese black dates, and lotus seeds. Drink 3 times daily.

Avoid: spicy, stimulating foods, overworking, obscene visual images, masturbation, sleeping on one's back (sleep on the side instead)

SORE THROAT (LARYNGITIS)

Sore throat can be caused by various factors including common cold, flu, eating too much spicy food, etc. There may also be a lot of mucus, fever and chills, headaches, and so on.

Recommendations: carrots, olives, daikon, celery, seaweed, licorice, dry unripe prunes, cilantro. Drink a lot of water.

Remedies:
1. Make tea from carrots and olives; drink 3 times daily for at least 1 week.
2. Make tea from daikon radish and green apples; drink 2 times daily.
3. Lightly cook seaweed, preserve with brown sugar for 3 days; eat daily for 1 week.
4. Make tea from cilantro, 1 T. green tea and a little salt, steeping for about 5 minutes.
5. Slowly chew and swallow rock sugar and cilantro.
6. For dry, hot throat, take a spoonful of honey in a glass of warm water, and drink.

Avoid: alcohol, smoking, pollution, sleeping with the mouth open, stimulating or spicy foods, fatty foods

157

STONES (GALL BLADDER, KIDNEY OR URINARY TRACT)

Various combinations of minerals can calcify or crystalize in the gallbladder, kidney, or urinary tract. These can range from the size of a grain of sand to 2 inches in diameter. Gallstones are a combination of bile and minerals and are characterized by pain in the right upper abdomen or pain in the corresponding area of the back and shooting up to the shoulder blade. Gallstones may also cause poor digestion of fats. If the gallstones obstruct the flow of bile, the result may be jaundice. Kidney stones are formed as the kidneys filter excessive minerals in an acid environment which combine with either excessive calcium or wastes in the blood. These are very painful, with the pain being in the kidney area of the lower back or the corresponding area on the front of the abdomen. There may also be painful urination with kidney stones.

Recommendations: cornsilk, water chestnuts, seaweed, beet tops, watermelon, celery, watercress, winter melon, pearl barley, walnuts, watermelon rind, winter melon rind, green tea powder, distilled water

Remedies:
1. Drink watermelon juice.
2. Drink celery, carrot, and water chestnut juice.
3. Drink cornsilk tea for water; 3-5 glasses daily.
4. Drink tea from beet tops, winter melon rind, and watermelon rind.
5. Take 2 teaspoons ground walnuts in cornsilk tea.
6. Take 1 teaspoon green tea powder in warm water 3 times daily.

Note: After consuming any of the above diuretic remedies, do some mild jumping exercise to help break up the stones.

Avoid: spicy foods, fried foods, oily foods, coffee, hard water, spinach, citrus, tomatoes, and spinach combined with tofu or dairy products

TINNITUS (EAR RINGING)

This is a common problem that has two major causes: The first is a local problem in which there may be a local obstruction or infection, nerve damage, drug interference, etc. The second stems more from a systemic condition such as coronary heart disease, hypertension, kidney weakness, etc. Along with ringing in the ears, one may also complain of headaches, irritability, restlessness, dizziness, red face, sore back, vomiting, nausea, etc.

Recommendations: black sesame, black beans, walnuts, grapes, celery, oyster shells, pearl barley, azuki beans, Chinese black dates, yams, lotus seeds, chestnuts, chrysanthemum. Get plenty of sleep, massage the neck and head area, and try to live in a quiet, peaceful place, if possible.

Remedies:
1. Make tea from lotus seeds and chrysanthemums.
2. Make juice from celery and grapes, drink 1 c. 2 - 3 times daily.
3. Cook azuki beans and black beans with rice porridge and eat at least once daily.
4. Boil Chinese black dates, walnuts, and lotus seeds with rice porridge and eat once daily.

Avoid: loud noise, stress, tension, stimulating foods, spicy foods, smoking, alcohol, coffee

ULCERS (STOMACH OR DUODENUM)

Ulcers can occur anywhere along the food pathway, from the mouth to the stomach to the intestines. Ulcers can also occur in the vagina. The most common place for ulcers to occur are the stomach and duodenum (first part of the small intestines). Ulcers are characterized by burning pain. In the stomach, pain is usually worse on an empty stomach; if the ulcer is further down, there will be pain after meals. There may also be nausea. If the stools are black (digested blood), the ulcer is higher than the stomach. If stools are red, the ulcer is lower than the stomach. If the blood is mixed in the stool, the ulcer is in the small intestines. If blood is on the stool then the ulcer is in the lower intestines or a result of a hemorrhoid.

Recommendations: potatoes, honey, cabbage, ginger, figs, papayas, squid bone, peanut oil, kale, persimmons

Remedies:
1. For mouth ulcers, apply the ash of charcoaled eggplant.
2. Drink potato juice daily on an empty stomach for at least 2 weeks.
3. Drink warm kale juice or cabbage juice on an empty stomach to help heal the ulcer.
4. Take 2 teaspoons peanut oil every morning on an empty stomach to help close the wound.
5. Drink fig juice.
6. Bake squid bone until crisp, powder it and take 1 teaspoon daily with honey.
7. Take blended papaya and milk or soy milk. Note, this remedy would not be good for a person with a lot of mucus, dampness, or allergies, unless soy milk were substituted for the milk.

8. Take 2 tablespoons steamed honey on an empty stomach in the mornings.
9. Cook ginger (an amount the size of the thumb) with rice and have for breakfast every morning on an empty stomach.
10. Dry and charcoal persimmon and grind into powder; take 1 T. in a glass of warm water.

Avoid: spicy foods, hot foods, stimulants, shellfish, coffee, smoking, alcohol, fried foods, and stress

WORMS

This is a common condition among children. It can manifest in such symptoms as decreased appetite, abdominal pain, nausea, diarrhea or constipation, vomiting, anal itching at night and malnourished appearance. There are many types of worms including roundworms, pinworms, tapeworms, hookworms, and other various intestinal worms.

Recommendations: pumpkin seeds, papaya seeds, coconut, garlic, hawthorn berries, sunflower seeds, prunes, ginger, vinegar, black pepper

Remedies:
1. Make tea from 10 unripe prunes, 6 g. black pepper and 3 slices fresh ginger. Drink 1 cup, twice, an hour apart in the morning on an empty stomach. Do this every day for 1 week.
2. Take raw 1 T. pumpkin seeds, ground to powder, with warm water, twice in the morning an hour apart, every day for 1 week.
3. Remove shells of sunflower seeds and eat 2 T. every morning on an empty stomach.
4. Make tea from hawthorn berries and betel nuts and drink 2 cups in the morning on an empty stomach, 1 hour apart.
5. Charcoal black pepper, grind to powder, take 1/2 t. 3 times daily with warm water.
6. Make tea from betel nut and pumpkin seeds. Eat pumpkin seeds then drink the tea and within about 4 - 5 hours expect diarrhea and excretion of the worms.
7. Take white part of green onion, make into juice and add 1 - 2 t. sesame oil; take 2 times daily on an empty stomach for 3 days.
8. Take coconut juice and 1/2 of a coconut every morning on an empty stomach; wait 3 hours before eating.

9. Take garlic on an empty stomach every morning.
10. Soak cotton with rice vinegar and plug up anus at night for three days, changing cotton each day. This will attract the worms to the anal area. Or do a rice vinegar enema and hold in all night; do this 3 days in a row.
11. Mash garlic and mix with vaseline, apply around anus every night for 3 days.
12. Mix raw garlic juice and rice vinegar with an equal part water and take on an empty stomach 3 days in a row.
13. Take 1 t. ground papaya seeds with warm water every morning on an empty stomach for 7 days.

Avoid: unsanitary foods, uncooked, raw foods

SECTION

Simple Vegetarian Recipes

SIMPLE, VEGETARIAN RECIPES

These recipes are provided to serve as a guide to those wishing to move away from a heavily meat-based diet. Ideally, meat should comprise no more than 1/10 of the diet. Soy foods such as tofu, tempeh, soy milk and wheat gluten can provide good alternatives to animal products.

Cooking is an art. To do it well one must be creative, paying attention to how the combinations look as well as how they taste. Always choose foods according to what is seasonally available. Feel free to make substitutions in the recipes with this in mind. Let your taste buds guide you in the appropriate seasonings and combinations of dishes.

Some of the recipes call for tamari. This is a naturally aged soy sauce. Miso is a salty, aged soybean and grain paste, used for seasoning. Also used for seasoning is Bragg's Liquid Aminos; this is a low salt soy liquid, available in health food stores. Kuzu and arrowroot are thickening agents, similar to cornstarch. Couscous is a grain product that comes from the heart of duram wheat and is sweet in flavor.

Many of the recipes use sea vegetables such as kombu, wakame, nori, or hiziki. Sea vegetables (also known as seaweeds) should be included in the diet regularly for they are an excellent source of nutrients, particularly the minerals. They are also known to alkalinize the body, purify the blood, help dissolve fat and mucus deposits, and neutralize radioactive matter. Seaweeds come in a wide variety of shapes and sizes. The thin sheets called nori can be used to wrap grains or vegetables. Wakame and kombu are good soup additions.

167

Kombu added to beans increases digestibility and decreases cooking time. One of the most flavorful sea vegetables is the red leafed dulse. The adventuresome may wish to try arame or hiziki; these look like thin black noodles, and are delicious with vegetables or tofu. Agar flakes can be used to make a gelatin-like dish called kanten. In general, sea vegetables (except nori) need to be rinsed and soaked prior to using. For soups, just washing is sufficient. Many of the seaweeds are easily available in oriental markets or health food stores.

In the recipes that follow, substitutions may need to be made to follow a specific remedial diet. For example, a person with Candida yeast infection should leave out the tamari and miso (fermented foods) and substitute herb salt or some other seasoning. Someone with a cold type condition may need to add more warming foods to the recipes, such as scallions, garlic, ginger, pepper, etc. Those with hot type conditions may need to leave out the warming foods, and so forth.

The following common abbreviations are used:
"t." is teaspoon
"T." is tablespoon
"c." is cup

SOUPS

Sweet Squash and Seaweed Soup

1 stalk celery, diced
1 butternut squash (or other winter squash)
A few chopped leaves of Chinese cabbage
A small onion or bunch of scallions
1 small piece of wakame seaweed

Begin with 2 quarts water. Simmer the winter
squash, peeled and diced, and the wakame, cut into
small pieces. Add the onion and celery pieces.
When the vegetables are tender, add 2 T. tamari
or Bragg's Liquid Aminos and 3 T. garbanzo miso (or
other light miso) which has been dissolved in a
small amount of broth. Garnish with a sprig of
cilantro. Serves 4.

Summer Vegetable Soup

1 onion
2 carrots
1 clove garlic
1 zucchini squash
2 tomatoes
1 handful green beans
1 cup fresh corn

Chop vegetables into small pieces; add to 2 quarts
water. Cook until tender then add 1 c. tomato
sauce, heat until warm. Season to taste with herb
salt, tamari, or Bragg's Liquid Aminos and garnish
with finely chopped cilantro and chives. Serves 4.

Soup Stock

4 6-8 inch pieces kombu seaweed
6 Chinese mushrooms
1 carrot
1 stalk celery
1 onion

Bring 2 quarts water to a boil with the above vegetables, then simmer for 1 hour. Strain and use the liquid for making soups or grains. It will store well in the refrigerator for about a week. Use the vegetables in some dish, perhaps a soup.

Black Bean Sauce or Soup

1 c. black beans
1 four inch piece kombu
1 small onion, finely chopped
2 garlic cloves
3 T. tamari
1 t. ginger juice
1/2 red bell pepper
2 T. cilantro

Soak beans overnight. Discard soak water, cover with fresh water and cook beans and kombu for about an hour. You may need to add more water. During the last 20 minutes of cooking, add garlic, onions, and red bell pepper. Mix tamari and ginger juice in at the end. Blend for a creamy sauce to pour over grains or steamed vegetables. Serves 4.

Beet Sauce or Soup

5-6 carrots

2-3 large beets
2 onions
2-4 stalks celery
2 T. miso
3-4 cloves garlic

Cook vegetables with 3-4 cups water until tender.
Blend vegetables with the cooking liquid. Add the
miso, 2 T. olive oil, 1 t. basil and 1 t. oregano,
and 1 t. umeboshi plum paste. Return to flame and
simmer for 20 minutes to mix flavors. For sauce,
add 2 T. arrowroot, cornstarch, or kuzu, dissolved
in 1/4 c. water to the mixture and heat until thick
and smooth. Serve sauce over noodles or steamed
vegetables. Serves 4-6.

Chinese Noodle Soup

8 Chinese mushrooms, soaked with stems removed and
  sliced very thin
6 white mushrooms, sliced very thin
1 red bell pepper, sliced very thin
1 small yellow squash, sliced
1 small piece wakame, sliced into small pieces

Put vegetables into 2 quarts water or vegetable
broth; cook until tender. Then add the following:
3 T. chopped cilantro
3 chopped green onions
1 T. tamari
1 t. peanut oil or toasted sesame oil
1 small handful bean threads (mung bean noodles)

Remove from fire and let sit, covered for 5
minutes. Serves 4.

Winter Melon Soup

3 qt. vegetable broth
3 c. chopped and peeled winter melon
2 carrots
2 celery stalks
1 onion
12 Chinese mushrooms, stems removed
6 oz. tofu noodles or finely sliced baked tofu

Cook together until tender, about 25 minutes. Then season with 1 t. chives, 1 T. tamari, and 1 t. peanut oil. Serves 4.

Creamy Split Pea Soup

1 c. green split peas
3 c. water
1 six inch piece kombu
1 carrot
1 celery stalk
1 small onion
1 t. tamari

Cook peas and kombu until soft. Add the vegetables and cook another 15 minutes. When vegetables are done, put in blender with the tamari, 1 T. cilantro, 1/4 t. paprika, 1/2 t. curry powder, 1/2 t. coriander seed powder, a pinch of nutmeg, and 1/2 c. almond or cashew milk. Serves 4-6.

GRAIN DISHES

Fancy Rice

Cook brown rice as usual with 2 c. water to 1 c.

172

dry rice. After about 25 minutes, add a finely
chopped carrot, 3 chopped scallions, and 1/4 red
bell pepper, finely chopped. Cook another 20
minutes or until water is all absorbed. Serves 2.

Nori Burritos

Toast sheets of nori seaweed briefly over the flame
until it changes color from brown to green (this
take about 15 seconds) or use "sushi nori" that has
already been toasted. On one end, lay out cooked
rice, chopped green onion, steamed carrot slices,
pickled ginger, and crushed, toasted sesame seeds.
Roll up like a burrito, moistening the edge to get
it to stick. The edge can be moistened with tamari
or Bragg's Liquid Aminos for added flavor.

Vegetable Pie

Crust: Cook 1 c. brown rice with 2 3/4 c. water
for 30 minutes, then add 1/2 c. couscous and cook
another 10-15 minutes or until water is absorbed.
When done, stir in the following:
1 c. grated jicama root
1 t. chives
1/2 t. basil
1/4 t. curry powder
1 t. tamari or Bragg's Liquid Aminos

Press into a pie pan and add the following, finely
chopped:
6 oz. tempeh
2 small carrots
1 leek
1 celery stalk
5 Chinese mushrooms, soaked with stems removed

Steam the pie for 30 minutes. Garnish the top with chopped cilantro. Serves 4-6.

Millet Patties

Cook 1 c. millet in 3 c. water for 30 minutes, or until water is absorbed. Add 1/2 t. basil, 3 finely chopped scallions, 1 T. tamari, and 1/4 c. grated carrot; mix well. Put 2 inch wide patties on an oiled cookie sheet and bake at 325 degrees for 20-30 minutes. They should be crisp on the outside. Serves 4-6.

Stuffed Pumpkin

Cut the top off a small pumpkin; clean out the seeds and strings; save the lid. Fill with the following mixture:
3 c. cooked rice or barley
1 T. crushed, toasted sesame seeds
2-3 stalks celery, sliced
1 onion, finely chopped
1 T. parsley
1 t. thyme
1 t. sage
1/2 t. rosemary
1 T. tamari

Cover with lid and bake at 350 degrees for 1 1/4-1 1/2 hours (until fork easily goes into pumpkin). Serves 4-6.

Simple Couscous Pie

1 c. couscous
1/4 c. amaranth or quinoa or millet (presoaked a

few hours)
1 1/2 c. boiling water or broth
6 Chinese mushrooms, soaked and sliced
1 c. winter squash, mashed or grated
1 small leek
2 chard leaves
1/2 red bell pepper

Soak grains in the water 15 - 30 minutes, until
soft. Mix with vegetables, all finely chopped.
Press into a pie pan and top with chopped walnuts.
Steam 40 minutes over medium flame. Serves 6.
Variations:
1. Substitute 1 c. fresh corn kernels for the yam.
2. Substitute 1 c. grated carrot for the squash.
3. Substitute 1 c. spinach for the chard.

This is an easily portable dish, good for lunch
packs.

Basic Protein Cereal

1 c. brown rice (or 1/2 barley, 1/2 brown rice)
1/3 c. soybeans
1 T. sesame or sunflower seeds

Soak above in 3 c. water overnight or in hot water
for a few hours. Pour into blender and blend well.
Pour into a bowl and steam for 1 1/2 to 2 hours.
Serves 4.

Variations:
1. Substitute black or azuki beans for the soybeans.
2. Substitute 1/2 c. millet for 1/2 c. rice.
3. Substitute walnuts or pecans for the sesames.
4. Season with ginger or cinnamon, or honey or
   rice syrup, or nut butter.

5. Substitute raw peanuts for the soybeans.

Chestnut Rice

1/2 c. dried chestnuts
1/3 c. raw peanuts
1 c. brown rice or sweet rice

Soak together the above with 3 3/4 c. water overnight or in hot water for several hours. Pour into a bowl and steam over low flame for 2 hours, stirring occasionally, until chestnuts are tender. Serves 4.

Variations:
1. Substitute walnuts for the chestnuts.
2. Substitute 1/2 c. barley for 1/2 c. rice.

Simple Grain Dish

1 c. whole grains (brown rice, barley, millet,
    sweet rice, couscous, or a mixture of these)
2 c. water

Mix grains and water and steam for 1 1/2 - 2 hours over a medium flame. Serves 2 - 4.

OR:
Use 1 c. grain to 2 - 2 1/2 c. water to cook grains directly over the flame (as opposed to steaming) for 45 - 50 minutes, or until the water is all absorbed.

Variations:
1. Add dates or raisins and cinnamon for seasoning.
2. Add steamed peanuts.
3. Add brown rice syrup or maple syrup.

The Fastest Cereal: Couscous

Pour 1 c. boiling water over 1 c. couscous. Let sit for 5 minutes, covered. Garnish with scallions and cilantro. Serves 2 - 4.

Variations:
1. Omit the scallions and cilantro and add a grated apple, 1/4 c. raisins, and a pinch of cinnamon.
2. Add steamed peanuts.
3. Add 1/2 c. grated carrots, and a pinch of ginger.

Steamed Corn Bread

1 c. grated apple (or chopped fresh pineapple)
2 c. coconut milk or soy milk or almond milk or
      pineapple-coconut juice
1 medium banana
1/3 c. whole wheat flour
1 c. cornmeal
1/2 c. oatmeal or millet flour or brown rice flour
1/4 c. raisins (optional)

Blend the liquid with the banana. Add the rest of the ingredients and mix well. Pour into a pie plate and steam 30 minutes over medium flame. It is done when chopstick inserted in the center comes out clean. Serves 6.

Variations:
1. Substitute 1 c. grated carrot for the apple or use 1/2 carrot and 1/2 apple.
2. Add a pinch of each cinnamon, ginger, and nutmeg.
3. Add 1/4 c. coconut.

The following recipe is reprinted courtesy of Lily Chuang from her cookbook, <u>Chinese Vegetarian Delights: Sugar and Dairy Free Cookbook</u>.

MOCHI
Serves 4-6

Soak 2 c. brown or black sweet rice in 2 c. water. Then put in blender, a little bit at a time. Continue until all is blended.

OR: Combine 2 c. powdered brown or black sweet rice and 2 c. water. Mix together well.

Steam for 1 1/2 hours on medium flame, covered. Open and stir well about 1/2 hour before it is done. Let the rice paste cool.

Wet hands to handle the rice paste. Form a small ball, flatten between hands, and put a small amount of one of the following fillings in the center: a combination of chopped, cooked Chinese mushrooms, seaweed, baked tofu, and seasoning; bean paste (azuki, black, or mung - good in summer); nut butter; or raisins. For a sweeter variety, fill with bean paste and honey or rice syrup; this makes an excellent dessert. Close the patty and form a ball. Roll in one of the following: coconut, sunflower meal, sesame meal, cashew meal, carob powder, or toasted soybean flour.

BEAN AND TOFU DISHES

Tofu and Mushroom Casserole

2 lb. plain tofu, lightly steamed
12 large Chinese mushrooms, soaked until soft,thin-
   ly sliced
2 c. pea pods
1 bunch scallions

Slice tofu into 1/2 inch slices and put in bottom
of rectangular baking dish. Lightly simmer
mushrooms then add pea pods and scallions for
last 5 minutes. Put these vegetables on top of the
tofu. Use the vegetable cooking water plus enough
water to make 3 c. liquid. Add 2 T. tamari or
Bragg's Liquid Aminos. Dissolve 3 T. kuzu,
arrowroot, or cornstarch in a small amount of
liquid; add to the rest of the liquid, simmer,
stirring often, until the liquid thickens. Pour
this gravy on top of the tofu and vegetable
mixture. Garnish with crushed, toasted almonds and
finely chopped cilantro.
Serves 4.

Azuki Bean and Squash Casserole

1 c. azuki beans, soaked overnight
2 6-8 inch pieces of kombu
1 small butternut squash or other winter squash

Cover beans and kombu with water and simmer about 1
hour, adding water if needed. Then add the cubed
and peeled squash. Cook until tender, about 1/2
hour. Stir in a pinch of sea salt or 1-2 teaspoons
tamari. Serves 4.

Clinton's Savory Azuki Beans with Chestnuts

1 c. azuki beans, soaked overnight
1/4 c. dried chestnuts, soaked 1 hour
4 six inch strips kombu seaweed
1 t. lycii berries (optional)

Soak azuki beans overnight; discard soak water.
Place kombu in pot then add chestnuts and beans.
Cover with 2 inches water and bring to a boil.
Simmer 2-3 hours, adding enough water to keep
beans covered. Add a pinch of sea salt or 1 t.
tamari and the lycii berries 10-15 minutes before
done cooking. Serves 4.

Tofu Skins and Mushrooms

Soak 12 strips of dried tofu skin (available in
Oriental grocery stores) and 6 Chinese mushrooms
in 4-6 cups water plus 2 T. tamari for at least 4
hours. Then tie each strip in a knot, and simmer
with the mushrooms, thinly sliced, for 20 minutes.
Add 8 sliced, white mushrooms and a sliced red bell
pepper and continue to simmer another 10-15
minutes. Pour off the liquid and thicken it with
1-2 T. kuzu or arrowroot (do this in a separate
pan, heating until thick). Pour the sauce over the
tofu and mushroom mixture and serve over steamed
greens. Serves 4.

Steamed Peanuts

Soak 1 c. raw peanuts in 2 c. water overnight
or in hot water for a few hours. Steam with soak
water for 1 1/2 - 2 hours over medium flame.
This makes a delicious, nutritious addition to
cereals, vegetable dishes, etc.

Scrambled Tofu

1/2 lb. tofu
2 stalks celery
6 white mushrooms
1 tomato

Chop vegetables finely. Saute in 1/4 c. water or
1 T. oil. When almost done, add crumbled tofu.
Let heat for 5 - 10 minutes. Season with 1 t.
tamari soy sauce.

Variations:
1. Substitute 1 beaten egg for 1/2 of the tofu.
2. Substitute 1 small zucchini squash for the
   mushrooms.

Tofu with Seaweed

1 package baked tofu, sliced or 1/2 lb. plain
   tofu, cubed
1 handful hiziki or arame seaweed, soaked in hot
   water 20 - 30 minutes
1 large carrot, diced
1/2 c. jicama, diced
1 small onion, chopped
4 Chinese mushrooms, presoaked and sliced

Stir fry carrots, onions, mushrooms then jicama in
small amount of water (or mushrooms soak water).
When almost done, add the tofu and seaweed. Cover
and let steam for 5 - 10 minutes. Season to taste
with tamari soy sauce and toasted sesame oil.

Variation:
1. Substitute wakame or kombu for the hiziki.
   Note these need to be presoaked for several
   hours.

181

2. Add diced burdock root (gobo) at the beginning with the carrots.
3. Use white mushrooms instead of the Chinese ones.

Tofu Dressing

1/2 lb. plain tofu
1/4 c. oil
1 T. lemon juice
1 t. honey or rice syrup
1 t. rice or apple cider vinegar
1/2 t. tamari soy sauce (or a pinch of salt)
1 T. sesame tahini

Blend until creamy. Use on salads, vegetables, or sandwiches.

Variations:
1. Add 1/4 c. poppy seeds.
2. Add 1 1/2 t. prepared mustard.
3. Add 1/2 t. basil and 1/4 t. garlic powder.
4. Add 2 whole green onions.

MISCELLANEOUS RECIPES

Sesame Seed Garnish

Wash 2 c. whole, brown sesame seeds. Toast in dry skillet, stirring often until seeds can be easily crushed between the fingers. Separately, heat 1/2 t. sea salt in dry skillet until the chlorine gas is removed (you will smell it). Then mix sesame seeds and salt and grind in blender or in mortar and pestle. Store in the refrigerator. Use on rice, vegetables, etc. The salt can be omitted if desired. Kelp powder may be substituted for the salt.

Basic Vegetable Stir Fry

Use a variety of vegetables, diced or sliced. Stir fry in a small amount of water or broth, covered, the slower cooking vegetables first (i.e. carrots, green beans, cauliflower, etc.), then add the faster cooking ones (i.e. jicama, zucchini squash, broccoli, etc.) When the last vegetables go in, you can add tofu or gluten pieces also. Presoaked seaweeds can be added near the beginning.

When everything is done, season to taste with oil, soy sauce (or Bragg's Liquid Aminos or herb salt) or your favorite cooking herbs. Basil and cilantro are particularly good with vegetables.

Variations:
1. Add steamed peanuts or almonds.
2. Add 1 clove of garlic at the beginning.
3. Add finely grated ginger toward the end of the cooking.
4. Add chopped green onions at the end.
5. Add Chinese mushrooms (presoaked) at the beginning.

Cashew Nut Stir Fry

1 small yam
1 small head cauliflower
1 leek or onion
2 summer squash
1 handful green beans
1/4 lb. white mushrooms

Chop vegetables into small pieces. Put in skillet with about 1/4 inch water. Cover and steam until vegetables are tender. Pour out any remaining water into a bowl. Add 1 T. arrowroot or cornstarch and stir until dissolved; pour back into vegetables and heat briefly until liquid thickens. Stir in 1/2-3/4 c. cashew nuts and 1/2 t. toasted sesame oil. Garnish with toasted sesame seeds. Serves 2-4.

Stir Fry Over Noodles

2 c. chopped broccoli
1 red bell pepper
2 garlic cloves
1 zucchini
2 leeks
1 carrot
5 white mushrooms

Heat 1 T. peanut oil; saute the garlic and leeks. Then add mushrooms, carrots, broccoli, and 1/4 c. water or broth. Cover and cook 5 minutes. Last add zucchini and red bell pepper and cook another 5 minutes. Season to taste with basil, cilantro, and tamari. Serve over whole wheat or rice noodles. Serves 2-4.

Almond Milk

Soak 1 c. raw almonds for at least 4 hours. Grind in blender with 2 c. water, strain and put the solids back in the blender and repeat the process 2 more times. Combining all of the strained "milk" there should be a total of 6 c. Put some of the liquid back in the blender with 1/2 t. vanilla or almond extract, a pinch of cinnamon, and 2 T. honey or maple syrup. Blend and mix back into the other liquid. Store in the refrigerator and use within a few days. Almond milk can also be sweetened by grinding in 5-6 dates or a small handful of raisins. This same procedure can be used to make cashew milk.

Soybean Milk

Soak 1 c. soybeans at least 8 hours, or as long as 3 days in the refrigerator. Blend with water, strain through a cloth, squeezing out the milk. Put the pulp back in the blender with more water and repeat the process until you have 2 quarts of soy milk. Bring to a boil and simmer for 15-20 minutes, stirring often to prevent sticking and boiling over. Soy milk can be used plain, mixed with carob powder and rice syrup, or blended with fruits such as papaya or banana (cool soy milk before mixing with fruit).

Protein Pudding

3 c. soy milk
1/3 c. rice syrup (or maple syrup)
1 bar agar seaweed

Rinse agar then mix with soy milk. Cook together until agar is dissolved. Mix in syrup. Pour into dishes and let firm.

Variations:
1. Add 1/2 c. raisins or chopped dates.
2. Add 1/2 c. pecans, sunflower seeds, walnuts, or cashews.

3. Flavor with 1/2 t. vanilla or 3 T. carob powder.
4. Substitute almond milk for the soy milk and garnish the top with 1/4 c. almonds when almost firm.

Pecan Pudding

2 c. soybean milk
1/2 c. pecans or walnuts
1/4 - 1/3 c. maple or brown rice syrup
3 T. arrowroot or kuzu or sweet rice flour
2 T. carob powder

Blend all ingredients well. Then heat over low flame until thickened, stirring constantly. Serve warm.

Wheat Gluten (Wheat Meat)

2 1/2 pounds gluten flour (or unbleached white flour or whole wheat flour)
1 quart water

Mix together to form a stiff dough. Then cover and let sit for one hour. Then put the bowl in the sink with the faucet on low and wash out the starch. Continue kneading the dough and pouring off the starchy white water until the water is clear. This will take many washings and much kneading (about 10 minutes). While washing the gluten, simmer the following broth: 2 quarts water, 3 small strips kombu seaweed, 1/3 c. tamari, 4 Chinese mushrooms and several slices of fresh ginger (onion, garlic, or bay leaf can also be used). When the broth has simmered 30 minutes, spoon out the solids. With the broth at a mild boil, drop in small (1") gluten pieces. When they

186

rise to the top they are done. The longer gluten cooks, the more tender it will become. For stronger flavored gluten, it can be marinated (soaked) in the seasoning broth for several hours after cooking. Gluten freezes well if you make a large batch. Gluten can be used whenever a "meaty" textured food is desired.

Basic Tomato Sauce

3 c. chopped tomatoes
1 bell pepper
1 garlic clove
1 small onion

Cook the above until tender. Then put in blender with 2 T. fresh basil or 1/2 T. dried basil, and 1/2 t. oregano, 1 t. onion powder, and 1 1/2 T. tamari. Return to pan when well blended.

Stir 2 T. arrowroot or cornstarch or kuzu into a small amount of water. Add to the tomato mixture, and heat, stirring often, until thick.

Variations:
1. Add 1/2 c. sauteed white mushrooms.
2. Add 1/2 c. zucchini.
3. Serve over noodles or steamed spagetti squash.

Simple Oil and Vinegar Dressing

Blend 1/2 c. each of oil and vinegar (rice or apple cider) or lemon juice and 1 T. tamari. You can also blend in 1/4 t. garlic or onion powder.

187

Sprouts

Sprouts are easy to grow and very nutritious.
The nutritional value of sprouts is increased
manyfold over the unsprouted seeds.

Rainbow Mix: This is a blend of azuki beans, mung
beans, and lentils. Soak seeds (together or
separately) overnight. Pour off the soak water and
rinse 2 times daily. A jar with a screen on top
is very handy for growing sprouts. Store in a
warm, dark place 3 - 5 days (remembering to rinse
twice daily). At the end of growth period, put in
sunlight for 30 - 60 minutes, for the leaves to
produce chlorophyll. These can be used raw or
lightly sauteed. Whole peas or whole wheat may
also be added to this mix.

Light Mix: This blend is alfalfa seeds, red clover
seeds, and daikon radish seeds (optional).
Sprout these in the same fashion as above. These
sprouts are used raw as a garnish for salads and
sandwiches.

Sandwich Fillings

These fillings can be used with any whole grain
bread or pita (pocket) breads or rolled inside of
whole wheat tortillas (chapatis).

1. Rainbow sprouts: Saute lightly in water or oil,
   mung, azuki and lentil sprouts, grated carrot,
   shredded red cabbage, soaked hiziki seaweed, and
   grated ginger.
2. Garbonzo spread: Cook garbonzo beans until soft
   then mash and mix with sesame tahini, lemon
   juice, garlic powder, and a pinch of salt.
   Garnish with alfalfa/clover sprouts and tomato

188

slices.

3. Nut butter: Almond butter, sesame butter, or cashew butter, grated carrots, green onions, and cilantro.

4. Soy burger: Combine cooked soy and garbonzo beans, grated carrots, sliced mushrooms and enough cornstarch or arrowroot or flour to hold together. Steam for 15 - 20 minutes over medium flame.

5. Sweet treat: Combine almond butter, rice syrup, grated apple, and a pinch of ginger or cinnamon.

6. Eggplant spread: Steam eggplant until soft. Mash and mix with sesame tahini, garlic, and lemon juice.

7. Colorful sandwich: Steam beets and carrots. Mash and mix with sauteed, finely chopped, tofu cabbage, and celery.

SECTION

Sample
Meal Plan

SAMPLE MEAL PLAN

Our meal plan is intended to provide some direction in nutritional meal planning. It is not meant to be a rigid regimen, rather a framework within which to plan your meals. Feel free to make substitutions to suit your needs. If your diet includes fish and meat, substitute for the tofu or other soy products up to 3 times a week. If your diet includes eggs or dairy products, those too could be substituted as protein sources.

In general, each meal should include a grain food. Breakfast should sustain us through the first portion of our productive day, so don't skimp there. Lunch is usually lighter because of the typical time frame within which we have to eat midday. Dinner time is usually more leisurely, and allows for more creativity in the kitchen.

For the Spring/Summer meals we will tend to eat lighter and include more fruits. Fall/Winter meals need to provide extra fuel to sustain our energy and keep us warm.

SPRING/SUMMER MEALS

	Breakfast	Lunch	Dinner
Monday	Cream of rice or wheat with raisins and cinnamon Steamed apples	Winter melon soup with tofu* Rice cake with nut butter	Stir fried vegetables with tofu and gluten* Brown rice*
Tuesday	Scrambled tofu with tomato and zucchini* Brown rice with pecans	Chinese noodle soup* Couscous with steamed peanuts* Papaya slices	Baked yam Tofu with seaweed* Fancy rice*
Wednesday	Apple/banana/carrot corn bread* Soy milk*	Fruit salad with soy yogurt and cashews Brown rice drink (amasake)	Tomato-mushroom sauce over whole wheat noodles and tempeh cubes* Steamed broccoli
Thursday	Couscous with grated apples and raisins* Almond milk*	Nori rolls with rice, steamed carrots and cilantro*	Vegetable tofu stir fry* Mochi rice balls*
Friday	Steamed pineapple corn bread* Almond Pudding*	Pita bread with rainbow sprouts and carrots* Green salad/ tofu dressing*	Tofu skins and mushrooms* Brown rice* Steamed eggplant
Saturday	Simple cereal with dates, raisins, and sunflower seeds*	Summer vegetable soup* Chapatis with avocado, sprouts	Couscous-corn pie* Green salad with sesame garnish*
Sunday	Scrambled tofu with egg* Couscous pie* Soy Milk*	Garbonzo spread on whole wheat bread* Apple slices	Vegetable stir fry* Protein cereal with peanuts and pecans*

Those foods that are marked by an asterisk (*) are listed in the recipe section with detailed instructions on preparation.

FALL/WINTER MEALS

	Breakfast	Lunch	Dinner
Monday	Basic protein cereal with azuki or black beans	Stir fry vegetables with tofu and seaweed*	Tofu skins with Chinese mushrooms*
	Steamed tofu with ginger, soy sauce, and nut meal	Simple grain dish*	Rice/barley/ couscous*
			Steamed broccoli
Tuesday	Simple cereal with dates, raisins, and peanuts*	Soyburger sandwich*	Couscous-corn pie*
	Steamed corn bread with sesame butter and rice syrup*	Vegetable soup*	Azuki beans and chestnuts*
			Steamed spinach
Wednesday	Simple cereal with ginger, scallions, miso, and seaweed*	Nori burritos*	Tofu-mushroom casserole*
		Black bean soup*	Stuffed pumpkin*
	Steamed broccoli and green beans		Pecan pudding*
	Soy milk*		
Thursday	Steamed corn bread with black bean paste and sliced banana*	Vegetable pie*	Cashew stir fry*
		Steamed greens	Millet and rice*
	Soy milk with carob*		Protein pudding*
Friday	Steamed corn, beets, and spinach	Stir fry vegetables over noodles*	Azuki bean and squash casserole*
	Pita bread sandwiches with mochi*		Sweet brown rice and couscous*
	Cinnamon soy milk*	Sweet squash and seaweed soup*	Cauliflower
Saturday	Simple cereal with tempeh, mushrooms, and celery*	Creamy split pea soup*	Beet sauce over noodles*
		Millet patties*	Tofu and Chinese mushrooms*
	Steamed apples		
Sunday	Chestnut rice with peanuts*	Chapatis with rainbow sprouts and carrots*	Black bean sauce over rice*
	Steamed carrots		Vegetable stir fry*
	Soy milk*	Steamed yam	

SECTION

Appendices

APPENDIX A

GLOSSARY

Astringent – substance that has a constricting action or causes contraction of orifices. Examples of astringent action are to stop sweating or stop diarrhea.

Arteriosclerosis – hardening of the arteries, usually due to aging or high consumption of fatty foods over a long period of time.

Ascites – accumulation of fluids in the abdomen, usually due to cirrhosis of the liver.

Carminative – substance that promotes normal flow of energy and removing obstructions; substance that relieves gas from the gastrointestinal tract.

Chi (Qi) – energy or life force, an entity that denotes the functional aspect of the body in Chinese Medicine.

Chi (Qi) Gong – a set of breathing exercises for strengthening and balancing the energy (chi), relaxing the mind, and for the purpose of maintaining health and curing disease.

Clears heat – to remove or neutralize pathogenic heat from the body; to soothe a hot, feverish condition with cooling foods or herbs.

Colitis – inflammation of the colon.

Cold-type condition – a condition caused by cold, one of the six pathogenic factors in the environment, or simply the result of not enough fire (yang) in the body. It is benefited by application of warmth (i.e. heating pad) or warming foods and herbs and aggravated by cold.

Cold-type person – one who tends to feel cold a lot, be pale-complexioned, lack energy, tend toward loose stools, not be thirsty, etc. (For a more thorough list of symptoms, refer to page 2 of text.)

Conjunctivitis – inflammation and infection of the mucous membranes of the eyelids as a result of too much heat in the body, specifically in the liver, according to Chinese Medicine.

Consolidate (the lungs) – to strengthen the lungs in conditions of chronic cough, asthma and short-ness of breath.

Cooling food – a food that has a counteracting effect to heat in the body, i.e., elicits a cooling response from the body; food of a yin nature; food that lowers metabolism.

Dampness – one of the external causes of disease that disturbs the normal flow of energy and particularly the digestive functioning of the spleen and stomach, characterized by heaviness, stagnation, and turbidity; fluid accumulation due to impaired water metabolism.

Deficiency – condition of weakness or lack of either energy or substance due to illness or improper lifestyle, diet, or mental attitude.

Descend – a method to move energy in a downward direction in the body.

Disharmony – imbalance or disease or lack of healthy function.

200

Diuresis – a process that promotes smooth urination and reduces edema.

Diuretic – a food or herb that promotes urination in order to relieve swelling or discomfort in urination.

Diaphoretic– a substance that induces perspiration in order to expel pathogenic factors and toxins.

Dryness – one of the six pathogenic factors in the environment. Disorder with dryness is associated with thirst, dry mouth and throat, fever, constipation, scanty concentrated urine, dry cough, emaciation, etc.

Dysentery – Extreme diarrhea and tenesmus due to bacterial or viral infection.

Dysuria – painful or difficult urination.

Edema – abnormal accumulation of fluids in the body; swelling.

Essence ("jing") – the source of life, found in eggs, sperms, marrow, and the brain and stored in the kidneys; provides for growth, development and reproduction throughout one's entire lifetime.

Five element theory – an ancient philosophical concept to explain the phenomena of energy transformation and the composition and relationships of the natural world and the human body. A further refinement of the concept of opposites (yin and yang) into four degrees, the fifth being the center or balance. (For a more thorough understanding of the five element theory, please refer to

<u>Tao, The Subtle Universal Law</u> by Ni, Hua-Ching.)

Gastritis – inflammation of the stomach.

Gruel (congee or porridge) – grain that has been cooked with extra water and cooking time to the point of being "soupy".

Harmonize – restore general balance; to bring together into smooth functioning.

Hot-type condition – condition that is usually caused by heat, one of the six pathogenic factors in the environment, or a lack of water (yin) to counterbalance the fire (yang) in the body. It is benefited by cooling foods and treatment, and aggravated by heat. This is usually an acute, excess condition, i.e., infections, fevers, boils, etc.

Hot-type person – one who tends to feel hot a lot, sweat freely, be red in face or tongue, have an excess of energy, be thirsty, etc. (For a more complete list of symptoms, refer to page 2 in the text.)

Hypertension – high blood pressure.

Jing – refer to "essence"

Lactostasis – hampered milk production or secretion due to physical or functional obstruction.

Leukorrhea – white or yellow mucous discharge from the cervix or the vagina.

Liver heat (or fire) rising – a condition in which an excessive amount of heat in the liver rises to the upper part of the body causing red painful

202

eyes, flushed cheeks, headache, fits of anger, emotional instability, dizziness, ringing in the ears, insomnia, etc.

Nephritis– inflammation of the kidney.

Neurasthenia – nervous exhaustion characterized by fatigue, weakness, headache, sweating, polyuria, tinnitus, dizziness, fear, photophobia, insomnia, etc.

Pathogen – a microorganism or substance capable of producing a disease. In Chinese Medicine it refers to anything that may cause imbalance within the body including environmental factors (wind, cold, heat, dampness, dryness, summer heat) and emotions.

Rebellious chi – energy that moves upwardly when it normally should be going down, i.e., coughing, vomiting, hiccupping, etc.

Shen – spirit.

Stagnancy – a sluggishness or impeded circulation of blood, energy, or body fluids.

Summer heat – one of the external causes of disease characterized by irritability, fever, headache, thirst, fidget, sweating, etc.

T'ai Chi Ch'uan – an ancient Chinese exercise for harmonizing the mind, body, and spirit, whose connected movements somewhat resemble a graceful dance.

Tonify – to strengthen or build.

Toxins – poisons; in Chinese Medicine this term

often refers to the presence of bacteria or virus.

Ventilate (lungs) – to disperse energy stagnation in the lungs and to soothe breathing and help relieve cough and asthma.

Visceras – internal organs.

Warming food – one that reduce coldness in the body or is of a yang nature; food that raises metabolism.

Wind – one of the external causes of diseases; a syndrome characterized by fever, chills, head and body ache. Internally, wind can also disrupt the balance manifesting such symptoms as dizziness, fainting, convulsions, tremor, numbness, or pain that moves around (like the wind).

Wind–cold – common cold or flu caused by the invasion of wind and cold. Symptoms are severe chills, mild fever, head and body ache, no sweat, sinus congestion, etc.

Wind–heat – common cold or flu caused by the invasion of wind and heat. Symptoms are high fever, mild chills, sore throat, body and head ache sweating, thirst, etc.

Yang – relating to the male, active, positive, firey, energetic side of life or nature of a person.

Yang deficiency – a lack of heat or fire (yang) within the body to counterbalance the water (yin), characterized by coldness, chi deficiency, tiredness, diarrhea with watery stools, etc.; a lack of energy to balance bodily substance.

Yin – relating to the female, passive, negative, watery, cool, substance side of life or nature of a person.

Yin deficiency – a lack of the coolness or water (yin) within the body to counterbalance the fire (yang), usually resulting in heat symptoms such as irritability, red cheeks, night sweats, insomnia, etc.; a lack of bodily substance to balance energy.

APPENDIX B

BIBLIOGRAPHY

For further reading on the subjects of Chinese medicine, nutrition, and health maintenance, the following books may be helpful.

Butt, Gary and Freena Bloomfield. Harmony Rules. London: Arrow Books, Ltd., 1985.

Colbin, Annemarie. Food and Healing. New York: Ballantine Books, 1986.

Essentials of Chinese Acupuncture. Beijing, China: Foreign Language Press, 1980.

Flaws, Bob and Honora Wolfe. Prince Wen Hui's Cook: Chinese Dietary Therapy. Brookline, Massachusetts: Paradigm Publications, 1983.

Gallagher, Paul B. "Chinese Herbal and Dietary Therapy". Yoga Journal, Issue 67 (March–April, 1986), 33–36.

Haas, Elson. Staying Healthy With the Seasons. Berkeley, California: Celestial Arts, 1981.

Jou, Tsung Hwa. The Tao of T'ai Chi Ch'uan: Way to Rejuvenation. Piscataway, New Jersey: T'ai Chi Foundation, 1983.

Kaptchuk, Ted J. The Web That Has No Weaver. New York: Congdon and Weed, 1983.

Leung, Albert Y. Chinese Herbal Remedies. New York: Universe Books, 1984.

Liu, Da. _Taoist Health Exercises Book_. New York: Perigee Books, 1983.

Lu, Henry C. _Chinese System of Food Cures_. New York: Sterling Publishing Co., 1986.

Lu, Henry C. _Doctors Manual of Chinese Medical Diet_. Vancouver, B.C.: Academy of Oriental Heritage, 1981.

Miller, Saul and Jo Anne. _Food for Thought_. Englewood Cliffs, New Jersey: Prentice-Hall, 1979.

Ni, Hua Ching. _8000 Years of Wisdom: Conversations With Taoist Master Ni, Hua Ching, Vol. 1_. Los Angeles: College of Tao and Traditional Chinese Healing, 1983.

Ni, Hua Ching. _Tao, The Subtle Universal Law and Integral Way of Life_. Los Angeles: College of Tao and Traditional Chinese Healing, 1985.

Pang, T.Y. _Chinese Herbal: An Introduction_. East Sound, Washington: T'ai Chi School of Philosophy and Art, 1982.

Teeguarden, Ron. _Chinese Tonic Herbs._ New York: Japan Publications, 1985.

Tierra, Michael. _The Way of Herbs_. New York: Washington Square Press, 1980.

The companion cookbook to The Tao of Nutrition comes highly recommended as the most healthful book of its kind available. It is written by the mother of one of the authors and utilizes the basic principles of diet discussed within. Unlike other Chinese vegetarian cookbooks, this one does not use sugar, dairy products, M.S.G., or frying:

Chuang, Lily. Chinese Vegetarian Delights: Sugar and Dairy Free Cookbook. Los Angeles: College of Tao and Traditional Chinese Healing, 1987.

For further recipes the following cookbooks may be useful. Substitutions may be needed in the Chinese vegetarian cookbooks which tend to use sugar or M.S.G. freely.

Colbin, Annemarie. The Book of Whole Meals. New York: Ballantine Books, 1983.

Estella, Mary. Natural Foods Cookbook: Vegetarian Dairy-Free Cuisine. New York: Japan Publications, 1985.

Fessler, Stella Lau. Chinese Meatless Cooking. New York: Signet Books, 1983.

Hagler, Louise. Tofu Cookery. Summertown, Tennessee: The Book Publishing Co., 1982.

Hoshijo, Kathy. Kathy Cooks Naturally. San Francisco: Harbor Publishing Co., 1981.

Lin, Florence. Florence Lin's Chinese Vegetarian Cookbook. Boulder, Colorado: Shambhala, 1983.

Lo, Kenneth H.C. Chinese Vegetarian Cooking.
   New York: Pantheon, 1974.

Shurtleff, William and Akiko Aoyagi. The Book of
   Tofu. Brookline, Massachusetts: Autumn Press,
   1975.

Weber, Marcea. Whole Meals. Newberry Park,
   California: Prism Press, 1983.

APPENDIX C

CHINESE FOOD SOURCES

Some of the foods mentioned for therapeutic use or in the recipe section are available only from an oriental market. Chinatown sections of any large city are sure to sell those foods. Many of the items can be obtained at the following stores:

LOS ANGELES AREA:
Al Hoa Supermarket
860 N. Hill St.
Los Angeles, CA.

Al Hoa Supermarket
7235 Reseda Blvd.
Reseda, CA.

Al Hoa Supermarket
421 N. Atlantic Blvd.
Monterey Park, CA.

Hong Kong Supermarket
717 New High St.
Los Angeles, CA.

Hong Kong Supermarket
127 N. Garfield Ave.
Monterey Park, CA.

Tak Shing Hong
835 B North Broadway
Los Angeles, CA.

Yee Sing Chong Co.
966 N. Hill St.
Los Angeles, CA.

SAN FRANCISCO AREA:
China Herbs and Native Products
622 Broadway
San Francisco, CA.

Chinese Grocery (mail order catalog available)
209 Post St.
San Francisco, CA.

Hong Kong Noodle Co.
847 Pacific Ave.
San Francisco, CA.

Mandarin Delights Market
1024 Stockton
San Francisco, CA.

Metropolitan Foods
633 Battery St.
San Francisco, CA.

NEW YORK AREA:
Down to Earth
33 Seventh Avenue
New York, N.Y.

Earth Harvest Trading Co.
700 Columbus Ave.
New York, N.Y.

Everything Natural
119 Montague St.
Brooklyn, N.Y.

The Health Nuts
825 and 1208 Second Ave.
Manhattan, N.Y.

The Health Nuts
2141 and 2609 Broadway
Manhattan, N.Y.

Integral Yoga Natural Foods
250 West 14th St.
New York, N.Y.

Whole Foods in Soho
117 Prince St.
New York, N.Y.

PHILADELPHIA AREA:
Arrowroot
834 Lancaster Pl.
Bryn Mawr, PA.

Essene
320 South St.
Philadelphia, PA.

Valley Health Foods
2571 Huntington Pl.
Huntington Valley, PA.

MIAMI AREA:
Touch of Nature
2829 Bird Ave.
Coconut Grove
Miami, FL.

Oak Feed Food Store
3030 Grand Ave.
Coconut Grove
Miami, FL.

CHICAGO AREA:
New City Market
1810 N. Halstead St.
Chicago, IL

INDEX

215

217

ear problems 38, 80, **144–145**
ears 16
eczema 44, 45, 50, 65, 69, **126**
edema (see also swelling) 7,
    28, 37, 47, 49, 50, 53, 59,
    71, 80, 81, 85, 87, 106, **127**
egg (see also chicken egg)
    14, 144
eggplant **37**, 114, 136, 141,
    149, 161
emotions 7, 15, 16, **17**, 20,
    100, 102, 106, 108, 121,
    130, 137, 145
energy 13, 14, 16
energy, erratic 16, 69
energy, low 7, 87, 108, 144,
    152
epilepsy 35
erysipelas 39
essence 14, 15, **201**
excess 19
exercise 17, 19, 20
external 17, 19
eye hemorrhage 79, 96
eye weakness 30, 31, 32, 79
eyes 12, 16, 35, 37, 43

fasting 19, 29, 55, 121
fear 16, 17
fennel 38, 60, 73, **91**, 123,
    140, 142, 152
fever 45, 46, 53, 94, 106,
    112, 116, 117, 145, 146, 157
fibroid tumor 47
fig **59–60**, 106, 107, 108, 118,
    123, 124, 132, 142, 153, 161
fish 65, 85, **86–87**, 120, 125,
    127, 132, 139, 144
fish bones caught in throat
    59, 94
five elements chart **10**
five elements correspondences
    chart **11**
five elements theory **8–12**, 14,
    201
flu 60, 61
fluid in the abdomen 71, 127
fluids, regenerates 55, 57,
    58, 59, 62, 646, 65, 66, 68,
    69, 70, 82, 93, 95
food poisoning (see also
    seafood or meat poisoning)
    80, 124
food retention 28, 29, 30, 35,

43, 48, 51, 70
frostbite 29, 31, 37, 61
frozen foods 22
fruits 23, **55–72**
fungus conditions 36, 37, 69,
    94

gall bladder 8, 9, 16
gall bladder, benefits 34, 75
gallstones 34, **158**
garlic 7, **37–38**, 87, 94, 95,
    101, 102, 103, 108, 109,
    110, 111, 115, 116, 120,
    123, 124, 127, 128, 130,
    133, 136, 137, 150, 151,
    154, 163, 164, 168
gas 50, 89
gas pains 91
gastritis 40, 61, **202**
general cleansing 29, 55,
ginger 7, 28, 33, 34, 36, 38,
    41, 44, 47, 551, 61, 74, 83,
    87, 89, **91**, 92, 94, 95, 101,
    102, 103, 109, 112, 113,
    114, 115, 116, 120, 123,
    124, 127, 130, 134, 140,
    144, 148, 151, 152, 156,
    161, 163, 168
ginseng 87, 120, 140, 156
glaucoma **129**
goiter 46, 47, 51, 57
goldenseal root 36
grapefruit 53, **61**, 118, 129
grapefruit peel **61**, 116, 148
grape **60–61**, 104, 112, 160
greasy food 18, 28, 128, 142,
    153
green bean **38–39**
green onion (see scallion)
gruel 39, 45, **202**
gum disease 94
gums, swollen 83

hardenings (see also tumors)
    46
harmonize 58, 92, **202**
hawthorn berry 9, 43, **62**, 91,
    120, 121, 124, 134, 136,
    137, 142, 152, 163
headache 12, 13, 44, 49, 83,
    110, 115, 116, 117, 129,
    130–131, 136, 139, 147, 148,
    149, 150, 151, 152, 157, 160
heart 8, 9, 14, 15

218

Books in English By Master Ni

New Publications
Internal Growth Through Tao - $13.95
Power of Natural Healing - $14.95
Essence of Universal Spirituality - $19.95
Guide to Inner Light - $12.95
Nurture Your Spirits - $12.95
The Key to Good Fortune: Refining Your Spirit - $12.95
Quest of Soul - $11.95
Eternal Light - $14.95
Attune Your Body with Dao-In - $14.95

Beginning Readings
Stepping Stones for Spiritual Success - $12.95
The Gentle Path of Spiritual Progress - $12.95
Spiritual Messages from a Buffalo Rider - $12.95
8,000 Years of Wisdom, Volume I and II - Each $12.50, *Both $22.00*

Taoist Classics and Esoteric Teachings
Book of Changes and Unchanging Truth - hardcover $35.00
The Complete Works of Lao Tzu - $12.95
The Taoist Inner View of the Universe - $14.95
Tao, the Subtle Universal Law - $7.50
Attaining Unlimited Life (Chuang Tzu) - paper $18.00, Hardcover $25.00
The Heavenly Way - $2.50
The Story of Two Kingdoms - hardcover, $14.00
Quest of Soul - $11.95
Eternal Light - $14.95

Personal Vision and Practical Development
The Uncharted Voyage Towards the Subtle Light - $14.50
Footsteps of the Mystical Child - $9.50
Workbook for Spiritual Development - $12.50
Poster of Master Lu, Tung Ping - $10.95; *with Workbook, $6.45 (2 shipping chgs.)*
The Way of Integral Life - paper $14.00, hardcover $20.00
Enlightenment: Mother of Spiritual Independence - paper, $12.50,
    hardcover $22.00

Materials on Taoist Health, Arts and Sciences

The Tao of Nutrition by Dr. Maoshing Ni - $14.50
Chinese Vegetarian Delights by Lily Chuang - $7.50
    -Set of Tao of Nutrition and Chinese Vegetarian Delights: $19.50
Chinese Herbology Made Easy by Dr. Maoshing Ni - $14.50
Crane Style Chi Gong Book by Dr. Daoshing Ni - $10.95

Videotapes
Attune Your Body with Dao-In (VHS) by Master Ni $59.95
T'ai Chi Chuan: An Appreciation (VHS) by Master Ni - $49.95
Crane Style Chi Gong (VHS) by Dr. Daoshing Ni - $65.95
Eight Treasures (VHS) by Dr. Maoshing Ni - $49.95
T'ai Chi Chuan I & II by Dr. Maoshing Ni - Each $49.95, Both $90.00

Audiotapes
Invocations: Health, Longevity & Healing a Broken Heart by Dr. Maoshing Ni - $8.95
Chi Gong for Stress Release by Dr. Maoshing Ni - $8.95
Chi Gong for Pain Management by Dr. Maoshing Ni - $8.95
Tao Teh Ching - $12.95, *Order the Complete Works of Lao Tzu and The Tao Teh Ching*
    audiotape set together: $23.00

How To Order

Name: _____

Address: _____

City: _____ State: _____ Zip: _____

Phone - Daytime: _____ Evening: _____

(We may telephone you if we have questions about your order.)

Qty.	Stock No.	Title/Description	Price Each	Total Price

Total amount for items ordered_____

Sales tax (CA residents only, 7%)_____

Shipping Charge (See below)_____

Total Amount Enclosed_____

Visa _____ Mastercard _____ Expiration Date _____

Card number:_____

Signature:_____

Shipping: In the US, we use UPS when possible. Please give full street address or nearest crossroads. All packages are insured at no extra charge. If shipping to more than one address, use separate shipping charges. Remember: 1 - 10 copies of Heavenly Way, Tao Teh Ching audio tapes and each book and tape are single items. Posters (up to 5 per tube) are a separate item. Please allow 2 - 4 weeks for US delivery and 6 - 10 weeks for foreign surface mail.

By Mail: Complete this form with payment (US funds only, No Foreign Postal Money Orders, please) and mail to: Union of Tao and Man, 117 Stonehaven Way, Los Angeles, CA 90049

Phone Orders: (213) 472-9970 - You may leave credit card orders anytime on our answering machine. Please speak clearly and remember to leave your full name and daytime phone number. We will call only if we have a question with your order, there is a delay or you specifically ask for phone confirmation.

Inquiries: If you have questions concerning your order, please refer to the date and invoice number on the top center of your invoice to help us locate your order swiftly.

Shipping Charges
Domestic Surface:	First item $ 3.25, each additional, add $ .50.
Canada Surface:	First item $ 3.25, each additional, add $1.00.
Canada Air:	First item $ 4.00, each additional, add $2.00
Foreign Surface:	First Item $ 3.50, each additional, add $2.00.
Foreign Air:	First item $12.00, each additional, add $7.00.

For the Trade: Wholesale orders may be placed direct to publisher, or with NewLeaf, BookPeople, The Distributors, Inland Books, GreatWay in US or DeepBooks in Europe.

Thank you for your order